ANXIETY

A Multidisciplinary Review

P TYRER

Imperial College School of Medicine at St Mary's,
London, UK

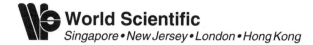

World Scientific
Singapore • New Jersey • London • Hong Kong

Published by

Imperial College Press
57 Shelton Street
Covent Garden
London WC2H 9HE

Distributed by

World Scientific Publishing Co. Pte. Ltd.
P O Box 128, Farrer Road, Singapore 912805
USA office: Suite 1B, 1060 Main Street, River Edge, NJ 07661
UK office: 57 Shelton Street, Covent Garden, London WC2H 9HE

British Library Cataloguing-in-Publication Data
A catalogue record for this book is available from the British Library.

ANXIETY: A MULTIDISCIPLINARY REVIEW

ISBN 1-86094-073-0

Printed in Singapore.

ANXIETY

A Mutidisciplinary Review

Dedicated to the tolerant tribe

Ann, illustrious illustrator
Clare, výborná učitelka
Freya, the human face of public health
Jonathan, man of many powers, and
Suki, organiser of manuscripts

PREFACE

Anxiety is a conundrum and our ignorance about its origins, generation, significance and purpose is profound. We certainly know much more about its manifestations but without this other information our interpretation of these could be badly flawed. Texts on anxiety often attempt to paper over these cracks and present a comprehensive picture of the subject, and although these are often internally consistent, they inevitably contain a great deal of speculation.

This is a personal account of anxiety in its many forms, encountered mainly in a pathological degree during thirty years of psychiatric practice. As such, it is bound to be idiosyncratic and somewhat deviates significantly from more conventional views, particularly with regard to classification. I have tried to be frank and honest about these differences, explaining the reasons for my concerns, and making it clear where my own views deviate significantly from the majority opinion.

Although there are sometimes specific reasons for these deviations, the fundamental one which crystallises my concern over existing views of anxiety is that the emotion has been excessively compartmentalised and its separate elements are too often studied in isolation. We need to be reminded that anxiety is one of the most prominent features of the psychiatric landscape. It is like an old and well recognised tree, that is visible from all perspectives, and whose roots penetrate deep into other conditions and cannot be considered in isolation. My personal view, and I am prepared to admit it may be a mistaken one, is that our present knowledge is so limited that we should continue to regard anxiety as a diffuse emotion that is rarely seen in pure form and that much of its significance in clinical practice and normal function lies in its interactions with other emotions and behaviour. The facts of anxiety are relatively straightforward; it is their content that confuses.

Despite these differences of opinion from those of others, the format of this book is a fairly standard one. The book is divided into two main sections, a general one in which the main features of anxiety are described, how it is measured and what physiological changes accompany it, and how it is interpreted in dynamic terms; and a second clinical section which describes the ways in which pathological anxiety is classified, how it is treated, and what are its usual outcomes. In a last chapter, I try to bring together the somewhat disparate elements of the preceding discussion to focus on the main core of pathological anxiety and how it relates to the other elements of the mood. There are many omissions, amongst which the most prominent may be the absence of significant discussion about the neuropharamacology of the subject, which I find bewildering in its speed of development and changes of emphasis, but which I am sure has contributed greatly to our understanding.

I have tried to write in relatively simple language but it is impossible to avoid discussing this subject in any depth without introducing the reader to a host of new words that now surround the subject. I have tried to give an appropriate explanation for each of these but appreciate that I may not be successful in clarifying all of them and apologise in advance; I do not understand them all fully either. Because I have indulged in a personal account I realise that many aspects of the subject may be under-represented and some other may be ignored altogether. What I hope will become apparent is that anxiety is both a healthy emotion and a major concern for a very large number of people and, for the latter, our efforts to reduce the suffering associated with it remain woefully inadequate. The book therefore attempts to illuminate our ignorance rather than offer easy solutions; it is in no way a self-help primer.

I should like to thank Jenny d'Souza, Jackie Reynolds and Sarah Dodd for secretarial help, and my many colleagues for giving me at least partial support for my aberrant views on this subject, among whom Nick Seivewright, Siobhan Murphy, Robert Kendell, Paul Pilkonis, Patricia

Casey, Brian Ferguson and Michael Stone are prominent. They have helped me to find a way of understanding the conundrum which I suspect is like the exhortation of the Irish priest, "the steep and narrow path between right and wrong", but at least has sustained me on my clinical and research travels.

Peter Tyrer   January, 1998

ACKNOWLEDGEMENTS

Acknowledgements following for permission to reproduce material in this book; the World Health Organisation and American Psychiatric Association, for diagnostic criteria for neurotic disorders from the *International Classification of Diseases* and the *Diagnostic and Statistical Manual for Mental Disorders*; Dr Philip Snaith for the Hospital Anxiety and Depression Scale, the Clinical Anxiety Scale and the Irritability, Depression and Anxiety Scale; the *Journal of Neurology, Neurosurgery and Psychiatry* for the Brief Anxiety Scale; Professors Isaac Marks and Andrew Mathews for the Fear Questionnaire and the Phobia Scale (Fig. 2.9); *Clinical Pharmacology and Therapeutics* for Fig. 2.11; *Psychological Medicine* for Fig. 4.6; Oxford University Press for Fig. 4.4, Professors Goldberg and Huxley and Tavistock/Routledge for Fig. 5.2; the *British Journal of Psychiatry* for Fig. 8.2; John Wiley & Sons for Table 9.5; and *Acta Psychiatrica Scandinavica* for Fig. 9.2.

CONTENTS

Chapter 1

WHAT IS ANXIETY?

What is anxiety? Let me count some of the ways in which it has been expressed to me over the past thirty years, mainly by people who have suffered greatly from it:

"it is like being about to die and never being able to leave that moment"

"being chased by dragons"

"worrying about every second of the future and always getting it wrong",

"it makes my body all a-jangle"

"indescribable awfulness"

"like an elastic band just about to break"

"like I've been injected with gun powder"

"not knowing who or what I am, just a feeling"

"like being at the end of the world and then the world never ends".

However, there is another sense in which anxiety is used in everyday life and this is not nearly so disturbing. People are anxious to get things done, to make sure things go well, to be on time for a big occasion and while awaiting a major event, whether it brings joy or sadness. It is when one comes across anxiety in this context that it becomes clear that anxiety is not something to be abhorred or stamped out; a world without anxiety would be a grey and boring place that would lead to frustration and torpor.

Anxiety therefore seems to cover a range of experiences, a large deal of which is normal and experienced by all at sometime in their lives, and some of which is pleasurable. At the more pathological extreme, anxiety becomes unpleasant, distressing and, in its most extreme form,

1

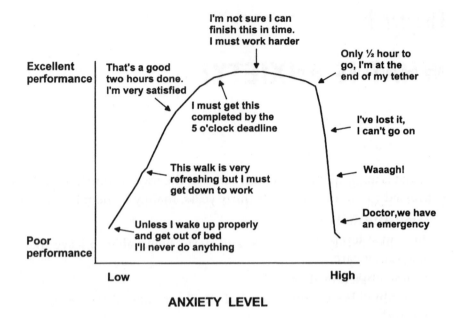

Fig. 1.1 The Yerkes-Dodson law of the relationship between anxiety and performance illustrated by an example.

one of the most intolerable experiences to which our minds and bodies are exposed. This range is best encapsulated by a research finding demonstrated by American psychologists 90 years ago. Yerkes and Dodson (1908) noted that anxiety had an unusual relationship to performance and this is best represented by an inverted U (Fig. 1.1).

The lowest level of anxiety is absolute calm, or more accurately described as deep sleep or, at an even more inactive state, coma. In such a state there is no response to most stimuli and only the most intense of experiences will arouse the individual. However, coma is generally an abnormal state and does not necessarily represent the total absence of anxiety. At somewhat higher levels the person is drowsy, often drifting in and out of sleep, and is functioning at a very low level. In Fig. 1.1, this person is at the bottom end of the U-shaped curve on the left. As awareness improves, performance and function also improve. The level of anxiety rises as basic drives need to be satisfied such as hunger, thirst, physical and sexual activities. In fact, at these levels anxiety is also a drive and is extremely important for the protection of the species.

As demands increase, anxiety does also, and is rewarded by an improvement in performance. Eventually, however, a plateau of activity is reached in which performance cannot improve anymore. In these circumstances the individual feels tense and anxious and under pressure but is able to cope with this without improving any further in performance. Once anxiety levels increase beyond this point, performance disintegrates rapidly. Concentration deteriorates, the ability to perform co-ordinated physical and mental activities is lost, and the person ceases to have any control over the task in hand. At its most extreme state the person returns to the primitive levels of activity found in the lowest levels of anxiety and (rarely) may need admission to an institution for care. The captions on each part of the figure indicate the subjective responses of an individual passing along this spectrum of "the rise and fall of the anxious man".

It is difficult to decide where anxiety is first noted on this spectrum. It is certainly not present early in the U-shaped curve and probably is only noted when each increment of demand no longer leads to an equal increment of performance and instead levels off towards the plateau. It is also uncertain from the above descriptions what the essential elements of anxiety are. Is it a feeling or a mood, a brain state, a syndrome of specific symptoms, particularly bodily ones, or a catastrophic interpretation of events? It is first necessary to define our terms.

THE ETYMOLOGY OF ANXIETY

Aubrey Lewis (1967), in a celebrated paper that demonstrates his breadth of scholarship, described the problems that can arise from different interpretations of the word "anxiety" and also showed that its etymological derivation covers all the elements of anxiety described above. The root of anxiety is the indogermanic word "Angh" which appears in Greek and Latin in a variety of words describing the feeling of constriction or throttling but also encompassing longer-lasting distress and discomfort. What is curious is that what is generally accepted as one of the richest languages in the world, English, has largely stuck to one word, anxiety, to describe both the acute and long-term forms of this feeling. This has led to considerable confusion as anxiety now has at least four separate meanings:

- a state of agitation and tension
- troubled in mind
- solicitous desire to effect some purpose (a use that will not be discussed elsewhere in this book as it is irrelevant to its subject)
- uneasiness about a coming event.

Table 1.1 The Words for the Two Forms of Anxiety in Different Languages

Language	Acute Anxiety (attacks) (associated with fear and bodily perturbations)	Chronic Anxiety (unpleasure, subjective discomfort, mental tension)
French	angoisse	anxiété
German	Angst	Erregungszustände
Italian	angoscia	ansieta
Spanish	angustia	ansiedad
Swedish	ångest	anxietas

Another word, anguish, used formerly to describe anxiety, has now been lost from the nomenclature as it has been transferred to the territory of depression, where it is associated with grief and despair. However, in other languages the distinction has been retained and there are usually two words for anxiety: one devoted to a long-term state which is equivalent to "troubled in mind" above, and another describing the acute episodes of anxiety in which there are bodily accompaniments such as tightness in the chest and difficulty in breathing, palpitations, sweating and tremor. Some of these words are shown in Table 1.1. Unfortunately, because of the all-pervading influence of English as a developing universal language, the separate meanings of these two words are in danger of being lost.

Table 1.2 Six Main Characteristics of Anxiety as a Morbid State (adapted from Lewis, 1967)

Descriptions of anxiety	Element	Best descriptive word (language)
Emotional state closely related to fear	Mood	Angst (German)
Unpleasant emotion	Anhedonia	Unlust (German)
Directed towards the future	Expectation	Furcht (German)
Absence of threat, or exaggeration of minor threat, despite intensity of emotion	Maladaptiveness	none available
Subjective bodily symptoms	Somatic anxiety	angoisse (French)
Objective bodily symptoms	Observed anxiety	none available

Lewis concluded from his review that there were six elements involved in anxiety and these, with some adaptation and abbreviation, are shown in Table 1.2. Anxiety is clearly a state of mood or emotion of which an excess is unpleasant; it is concerned with uncertainty and is directed towards the future rather than the past (and thereby differs importantly from depression). In its pathological form it represents an over-reaction to a threat which is perceived as greater than it really is. It is also associated with bodily accompaniments which are both experienced subjectively by the sufferer and can be observed, with varying degrees of accuracy, by other people.

One word which was conspicuously absent in Lewis' review was "panic". This may surprise any reader who is aware of contemporary writings on anxiety. Although the concept of panic is well described in early writings on anxiety, most notably by Hecker (1893) and Sigmund Freud (1895) in their description of anxiety attacks (Angstzustand), it was regarded as an integral part of anxiety neurosis (Angstneurose). Following the work of Donald Klein in the 1960s (described in more detail in Chapter 5), the concept of panic as a separate component of anxiety has become so well developed that it is now regarded as a completely different disorder. It is tempting to conclude from examination of the terminology of anxiety that if the two essential components of pathological anxiety (acute attacks and chronic inquietude) had been retained in English as well as in other languages, then the notion of panic as a separate condition would never have arisen.

Another word intimately associated with anxiety is fear. Fear is a special type of anxiety specifically associated with an object or setting; it is usually situational anxiety. Fear differs from most other forms of anxiety in that it is related to an external threat, whereas much of the rest of anxiety is either linked to an internal threat (the ferment and torment of one's own psyche) or is unfocussed. Persistent fears of situations naturally leads to avoidance of such situations, and the combination of fear and avoidance creates phobic anxiety, usually abbreviated to phobia.

Stress is another word commonly linked to anxiety. It is the most confusing word of all those used to describe anxiety. In Paris in the 1980s most of the benzodiazepine tranquillising drugs prescribed for the population were for "le stress" (Boyer, personal communication), yet the average patient with anxious symptoms blames stress for their cause; private clinics give special treatments for "stress anxiety"; and explanations for curious behaviour often argue that the individual concerned "had been stressed" at the time. Stress is therefore, apparently simultaneously, both a cause of stress and its consequence, a qualifying adjective and a passive verb. "What explanation have you for this sorry course of actions?", asked the judge. "Stress", my lord, says the anxiety-ridden prisoner, "I was stressed by the stress of it and I suffer from stress". When "distress" is introduced into this vocabulary, it can be exchanged with "stress" almost willy-nilly and this confuses the vocabulary further. Let us confine stress to its technical psychiatric use in the rest of this book, a word which is short for "stressor", an event or act that creates anxiety.

TYPES OF ANXIOUS REACTIONS

Already we have a set of terms which describe different forms of anxiety and we can now set them into context. It is first necessary to separate normal from pathological anxiety. This can be done quite easily from the Yerkes-Dodson curve in Fig. 1.1. When anxiety is promoting performance, it is essentially normal (the first limb of the U), and when it leads to a catastrophic loss of performance, it is clearly pathological (the second limb of the U). In between (the plateau phase), it is not quite clear when the anxiety becomes pathological. Before performance deteriorates, the sufferer may have a range of psychological and bodily symptoms — nervous and muscular tension, distractibility, palpitations, difficulty in breathing, tremor, headache — and when these become unpleasantly pervasive, the anxiety is clearly pathological.

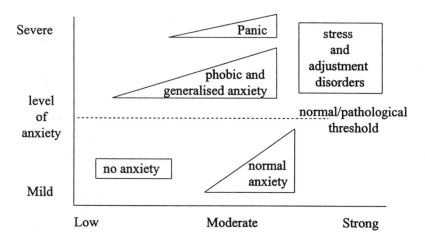

Fig. 1.2 Relationship between stress and anxiety disorder.

In Fig. 1.2 the different forms of anxiety that form the main subject of this book are shown in relationship to the intensity of stimulus (or level of stressor). At low levels of stimulus, most people do not have any symptoms of anxiety but a minority will experience pathological anxiety in various forms. The most severe of these is panic, sudden and unpredictable attacks of anxiety that are all the more distressing because they are so unexpected. Generalised and phobic anxiety (or unfocused and situational anxiety) are less severe, but it is still unpleasant and can also occur against a background of little stimulus. However, they are more common when the level of stress rises and this explains the triangular expansion in Fig. 1.2 with these disorders.

At somewhat more severe levels of stimulus, normal anxiety is experienced by most people. The psychological and bodily symptoms described above are present to some degree but are usually tolerated quite well as the source of anxiety is clear. In most instances, it is predictable when the stimulus will end, or what can be done to bring it to an end, and this helps to make the symptoms more tolerable. At more severe levels of stimulus, this ability to cope is suddenly lost and the formerly phlegmatic "normal" individual suddenly crosses the threshold to pathological anxiety and shows the disintegration of the second limb of the Yerkes-Dodson U. People in this group are suffering from stress and adjustment disorders, one of the psychiatric disorders with a generally good outcome, as once the stressor is removed there is a strong chance that normal nonanxious service can be resumed.

The main message from Fig. 1.2 is that all of us can suffer from anxiety disorders. "One touch of nature makes the whole world kin", wrote Shakespeare in reference to time, but he could equally have referred to anxiety. If the time and situation is right, we can all suffer the same attacks of panic, anxiety and fear than our less fortunate fellow-beings who have lower thresholds for suffering and tend to be labelled as "neurotic" misfits as well. The only time the neurotically anxious have the edge is when the level of stress is so great that all "normal" people go to pieces. For example, when a cluster of German bombs landed on St Thomas's Hospital in London in 1941, the psychiatric unit for neurotic patients was in the middle of the conflagration that followed. Amidst the scenes of panic that followed, it was observed that the most fearless of the rescuers of the patients in the main hospital were some of the most anxious psychiatric patients (Sargant, personal communication). When asked to explain this apparently unexpected ability to cope in the face of such obvious danger, one replied, "We feel like this (very anxious) almost all the time but don't know the cause. When the bombs landed we knew what the cause was and what we had to do; it was nice to have a reason for being anxious for a change".

WHAT IS THE CAUSE OF ANXIETY DISORDERS?

The reasons for the distinction between people who usually experience normal anxiety or stress and adjustment disorders only, and those who have more severe anxiety, is dependent on many different factors. Sometimes the phrase "dependent on many different factors" means we do not have a clue, but in this case it is an exact description. Both environmental and genetic factors are relevant at different times. Environmental influences on anxiety can begin early in life. Even difficulties experienced during pregnancy can contribute towards anxiety and problems in a child. For example, an Australian study of 143 low risk pregnant women expecting their first baby examined "the contribution of a woman's perception of her own childhood experiences, her trait anxiety level, socioeconomic status, and social support network" to subsequent problems in her relationship with her baby during the baby's first year. The first interview was carried out while the women were in their pregnancy, and two more interviews were carried out 3 and 12 months after the birth. The women who perceived their social network as less supportive during pregnancy were significantly more likely to describe difficulties in their relationships with their babies (Adler et al., 1991).

Of course, it is difficult to know whether the difficulties experienced here are a consequence of problems in the mother or the child. Most authorities would veer towards the mother being the major cause in this setting, but at another level it does not really matter. The developing child has two main people from which to draw experiences, mother and father, and if either of these shows evidence of anxiety or other difficulties that can affect relationships, they can easily be transferred to the child by a process (predictably) called modelling (Bandura, 1969).

Negative experiences model negative outcomes with respect to anxiety disorders. Brown and his colleagues (Brown and Harris, 1993; Brown *et al.*, 1993), in a study that could suffer from retrospective distortion, found that adverse experiences in childhood and adolescence (particularly parental indifference, sexual and physical abuse) increased the risk of both depression and anxiety conditions (but not mild agoraphobia and simple phobia) in adult life. For adult, anxiety disorders early adverse experiences appeared to be more important than indepressive ones. (This does not mean that later experiences, particularly major life events, are not important also in creating adult conditions, but the general view is that vulnerability is increased by negative early experiences.

The hereditability of anxiety is also relevant here. There seems little doubt that anxiety is inherited, but in what form it is, is an entirely another matter. Increasingly in genetics it has become apparent that the methods of "old genetics", simple twin studies identifying a single gene (e.g. the autosomal dominant gene of Huntington's chorea) are not particularly useful in the analysis of genetic factors in common conditions such as anxiety. As methods of genetic analysis become increasingly easy to carry out, there is little doubt that several genes will be discovered shortly that have an influence on anxiety.

The evidence to date is somewhat conflicting. Some studies suggest that anxiety has a stronger degree of hereditability than depression and other neurotic traits (Young *et al.*, 1971), but others suggest that depression and anxiety are inherited by the same mechanism. For example, in a study of 1033 pairs of female same-sex twins, the familial environment was unimportant with regard to cause, but genetic factors were important and shared for both major depression and generalised anxiety disorder (Kendler *et al.*, 1992). The authors therefore concluded that "the liability to major depression and generalised anxiety disorder is influenced by the same genetic factors, so that whether a vulnerable woman develops major depression or generalised anxiety disorder is a result of her environmental experiences". In the same group, a second study by Kendler and his colleagues (1995) suggested that two anxiety disorders, phobias and panic disorder (together with bulimia nervosa) are explained by one genetic factor and major depression and generalised anxiety disorder by another. Similar conclusions were reached in an Australian study (Jardine *et al.*, 1984).

HOW DOES ANXIETY DEVELOP?

Throughout this book a distinction will be made between normal and pathological (abnormal) anxiety. This is based essentially on the Yerkes-Dodson curve in Fig. 1.1, but it is useful to look at the actual psychological changes during the experience of anxiety and what happens to make it pathological (Fig. 1.3).

The initiation of anxiety is the awareness of threat. At very mild levels of anxiety, the word "threat" may be a little strong, but it indicates some degree of uncertainty that has a negative option attached. We all love to be in the state of uncertainty when all the options are pleasurable (witness the reactions of young children immediately before the opening of Christmas presents), but when just one is unpleasurable, anxiety arrives on the scene. If the negative possibility is removed, avoided or solved in some way then the anxiety disappears; these ways of dealing with anxiety all come within the normal range and are illustrated in stages 1 and 2 in Fig. 1.3.

If the cause remains unresolved the symptoms of anxiety, both psychological and physical, persist and in time tend to reinforce each other to create more anxiety. And, when this reaches a certain level, function begins to be impaired (this is the rocky road downwards on the Yerkes-Dodson curve). The sufferer cannot cope and, if no obvious help is available, may turn to alcohol or other available drugs to relieve symptoms, indulge in maladaptive avoidance of situations that create anxiety (the development of phobias), or somatise (i.e. assume the condition has a physical cause) and thereby deny the psychological symptoms of anxiety and its causation. These three elements are shown in stages 3, 4 and 5 in Fig. 1.3 and together these comprise pathological anxiety. Some kind of external intervention is needed at these stages and the responsibilities of clinical care begin here.

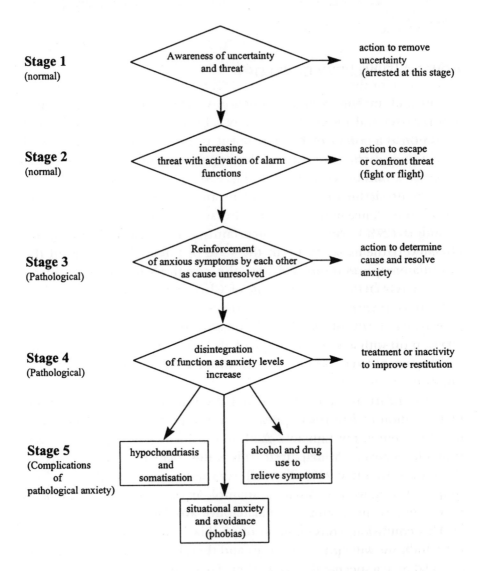

Fig. 1.3 The five stages of development of anxiety.

HOW COMMON IS ANXIETY?

Anxiety is one of the most common symptoms of ill-health and probably exceeds all others. This has always been suspected but has recently been confirmed in national epidemiological surveys. Such surveys attempt to examine a random sample of all people in the population for the condition under enquiry and, through sophisticated methods of analysis, are able to make allowances for non-responders and refusers and come up with accurate figures of the extent of the condition at a point in time (prevalence).

In a study carried out between 1993 and 1994 in the United Kingdom of 10,000 adults between ages of 16 and 64, no fewer than one in seven had a neurotic health problem in the week prior to interview, with a greater prevalence in women (ratio female/male 11/6). The symptoms of fatigue (27%), sleep problems (25%), irritability (22%) and worry (20%) were the most common symptoms. In terms of formal diagnosis, mixed anxiety and depression disorder (7%) and generalised anxiety disorder (GAD)(3%) were the most common (Meltzer *et al.*, 1994).

Similar findings have been found in the United States, with approximately 7% of people having an anxiety disorder (Regier *et al.*, 1990), most with generalised anxiety but 1–2% having panic symptoms. It is important to realise that the diagnoses of anxiety disorders, despite our best efforts to give them separate validity, overlap enormously with other conditions, particularly other anxious ones, and so the identification of one disorder almost always identifies another which, if not present at the time of assessment, will be before long. Thus, for example, Brawman-Mintzer *et al.* (1993) found in a study of generalised anxiety disorder that 23% of all patients had social phobia and 21% had simple phobia, with no less than 42% having had an episode of major depression during their lifetime.

This confusion, conveniently formalised in the term "comorbidity" (of which we will hear more later in this book), illustrates that the exact label of a specific anxiety problem is of relatively little value unless the degree of overlap with other conditions is specified very clearly. Rather than get bogged down in detail, it is reasonable to conclude that around 10% of the population have an anxiety disorder of some sort at any one time, and by any standards this number is enormous, amounting to 4 million people in the United Kingdom alone.

Much of this will get better spontaneously in the shorter or longer term: some indicates the early development of a more serious disorder while other conditions will produce relatively little handicap. Yet there are others which will be almost incapacitating; while some are so much an intrinsic part of the person's functioning that they are permanent components of the personality. Finding out where someone's anxiety belongs in this jungle is not easy; the rest of this book attempt to be a faithful guide.

Chapter 2

MEASUREMENT OF ANXIETY

The well known psychiatrist, Bob Spitzer, probably the main architect of our current systems of psychiatric classification, has an axiom which lies at the heart of his work — "if it exists it can be measured". Anxiety clearly does exist but is more difficult to measure than might at first appear. Although anxiety has many bodily and psychological accompaniments, it is fundamentally an emotion and can only be measured adequately by asking a person how he or she feels. This simple fact in an age of high technology may seem to some to be a big let-down, a failure of science. When neuropsychologists are able to detect minor variations in blood flow to different parts of the brain only a few millimetres apart, it must surely be possible to measure anxiety by something more sophisticated than a series of questions whose responses can never be recorded with the rigour of the other measurements of science?

Unfortunately, or fortunately for those who still value human discourse as a measure of communication, anxiety cannot yet be recorded objectively. All the physiological and psychological measures of anxiety discussed elsewhere in this book remain, at best, loose associations; they cannot be regarded as independent measurements of anxiety. That is partly related to the concept of arousal — high levels of physiological and psychological activity are associated with many states of emotion, not just anxiety — but also to the subtlety of emotional expression. When one considers how quickly pleasurable excitement can change to uncertainty, anxiety and panic with virtually no provocation, it would take a very sensitive measure to detect the changes and still be a suitable index of emotional state. This does not mean that such a measure is beyond us; it is just that our interpretation of the myriad of changes manifest in the central nervous system at any one time is beyond our comprehension and capacity to measure. When the great neurophysiologist, Sherrington, referred to the brain as "a giant loom" where "millions of flashing shuttles weave a dissolving pattern, always a meaningful pattern but never an abiding one", he emphasised the immensity of effort involved in interpreting complex behaviour and emotions, but nonetheless still hinted at their ultimate solubility. According to Spitzer's axiom, anxiety can be measured directly and probably without the need for questionnaires or interviews, but this is some way off. It is likely that such a measure would eventually come from the dynamic interpretation of neurotransmission in the brain which, in the last resort, must represent emotional states.

While we await this important advance, we must rely on questions and answers to elicit the symptoms of anxiety. This may either be in the form of standard (self-rated) questionnaires or as observer-rated instruments. As we are trying to record the subject symptoms of anxiety, the questionnaire format could be regarded as the most appropriate one. After all, an assessor is only able to elicit a small fraction of the "anxiousness" of an individual through observation, except when the subject is in a state of absolute terror, when all the sign of distress are obvious even to the untutored eye. However, if someone is having their level of anxiety monitored over a long period, say over two to four weeks, then it is sometimes difficult to disentangle present anxiety from that experienced in the recent past and this is a constant problem which may sometimes lead to observer ratings being preferred.

SOURCES OF ERROR IN QUESTIONNAIRES AND RATING SCALES

Accuracy in the measurement of anxiety can be obscured by common sources of error which apply to almost all questionnaire and rating scales. These will vary across situations but it is important to realise at the outset that anxious people tend, in general, to be influenced more than other people by these sources. Many of these errors are anticipated by constructors of these scales, but potential investigators should also be aware of them if they are to obtain reliable and valid data. An important source of error that is particularly common in rating scales is that some subjects tend always to agree or to disagree with the questions asked, a tendency known as the response set. This may also affect the general way in which some people complete rating scales and questionnaires. Some subjects always avoid extreme responses whereas others avoid "middle" responses. It is impossible to avoid these tendencies, bias towards the extreme and bias towards the centre, but they can be lessened by careful instructions.

Social desirability (social acceptability) describes the tendency to choose responses that the subject believes are either socially acceptable or desired or expected by the interviewer. Interestingly, anxiety is a respectable symptom (see Chapter 3) and tends therefore to be regarded as socially desirable and sometimes over-rated. The same may apply to response to treatment. The placebo effect, the positive response to a treatment that the subject regards as powerful but which is, in fact, a useless dummy, is also to some extent influenced by social desirability. Social desirability is often said to be reduced by inclusion of lie scales, which ask questions that select the responses that are socially desirable but which, on careful reflection, are highly unlikely to be true. The best known example of the lie scale is in the Eysenck Personality Questionnaire; it is an ingenious way around the problem but is not really a solution. Another way of reducing the effects of social desirability is the forced-choice technique, an approach that makes the subject choose from at two or more items which all have an equal degree of social desirability so are all of equal acceptability (or unacceptability).

Two other sources of error are particularly associated with rating scales. The halo effect describes a source of error in which the subject or observer scores all items according to existing prejudices or preconceptions. Some of these prejudices can be overcome. For example, the tendency to score the first item of a questionnaire because this fits either recovery or severe symptoms, can be overcome by making some of the responses negatively focused, so that the first-rated scores refer to severe symptoms, and others positively focused, so that the first-rated refer to absence of symptoms. This also ensures that the questions are read more carefully before the response is made. Another source of error in treatment studies, very common in anxiety, is the Hawthorne effect, the tendency of subjects involved in research studies to improve independently of any effects of treatment, as the increased attention and excitement associated with research involvement leads to a spurious improvement that can be interpreted misleadlingly.

The choice of questionnaires or observer ratings to measure anxiety is represented in Fig. 2.1. If the aim of the assessment is to find out the level of anxiety at a particular point in time (e.g. immediately before jumping out of an aeroplane on a parachute jump (a common choice of investigators wishing to measure high anxiety), then a questionnaire method or the same technique in its simplest form, the analog scale, is the method of choice. If the measurement is concerned with a specific form of pathological anxiety: generalised anxiety, panic or phobic disorder, then it may be appropriate to use a rating scale for generalised anxiety (focusing on longstanding background anxious symptoms), panic (focusing on the frequency and severity of panic attacks), or phobias (focusing on fear and avoidance in roughly equal

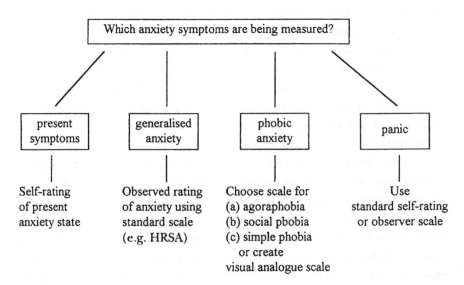

Fig. 2.1 Choice of measurement in anxiety.

degree). However, any attempt to constrict measurement to one set of symptoms only could be of limited value unless the specific hypothesis being tested in the measurement framework is similarly focused. It is therefore valuable to have a global all-purpose anxiety measurement as well as specific measures.

ANALOG RATING SCALE

The analog rating scale is a way of introducing the full range of anxiety (or indeed any other psychological measure) into a single record. This is represented by a line, commonly of ten centimetres in length, which is used to represent the range between no anxiety and the most extreme anxiety that has ever been experienced (Fig. 2.2). The scoring system for the visual analog scale, commonly abbreviated to VAS, is quite simple. The distance between the end of the left hand line and the mark is scored in an appropriate way (it is common to measure this to the nearest millimetre, as although this may give an impression of false accuracy, it is always a good policy never to simplify data in advance of analysis) and it is then scored accordingly. The big advantage of the VAS scale is that it can be scored quickly within a few seconds and therefore can be repeated many times. It is therefore particularly useful when recording anxiety over a long period or when measures have to be given many times during the course of each hour.

Its disadvantage is that some people find it hard to choose an appropriate point on the line if there are no anchor points and, as mentioned above, may tend to indulge habitually in scores at the ends of the lines (extreme-scorers), or alternatively, near the middle (middle-scorers). On the positive side, however, it is difficult on a ten centimetre line to decide at which point it is socially desirable to score it. Analysis of the data may sometimes be difficult because normal distribution is less common than skewed distribution of data and so transformation of the data (e.g. adding one and taking the square root, logarithmic conversion) may be necessary to allow parametric statistics to be used in the analysis.

Please mark how anxious you are at this moment by putting a mark across the line at the appropriate point. Remember the line represents the full range of anxiety

Presentation of scale

Absolutely	The most severe
no anxiety	anxiety I have
whatsoever	ever experienced

Marking of line

Absolutely	The most severe
no anxiety	anxiety I have
whatsoever	ever experienced

Scoring of response

52
mms

Absolutely	The most severe	Score
no anxiety	anxiety I have	52
whatsoever	ever experienced	

Fig. 2.2 Example of use of visual analog scale in recording anxiety.

The VAS is also less useful when comparing between individuals because of differences in perceptions in anxiety. Thus "the most severe anxiety I have ever experienced" for one person may be much more severe than in another and yet both could have the same score on the VAS. If the assessments are being made and analysed for one individual (and it is important to realise that over 1000 records per individual can be obtained relatively easily using the VAS approach), all these criticisms become much more muted.

SPIELBERGER STATE/TRAIT ANXIETY INVENTORY

This popular scale developed thirty years ago (Spielberger *et al.*, 1968) measures both present anxiety (state anxiety) and the general trait of anxiousness by recording the answers to twenty statements which are each scored on a four point scale. Thus, for example, the statement "I feel tense" has four possible responses from "not at all" to "very much so". The scale is extremely popular in experimental studies of anxiety but somewhat less so in clinical populations.

HOSPITAL ANXIETY AND DEPRESSION SCALE (HADS)

This scale, although relatively recent in development (Zigmond and Snaith, 1983), has become greatly used in the last ten years. It consists of 14 questions, half referring to anxiety (HADS-A) and half to depression (HADS-D), each scored on a four-point scale, so that a maximum score of 21 is obtainable for both anxiety and depression (Fig. 2.3). It was developed specifically for use in general hospital patients and the questions were chosen so that they did not overlap with the symptoms of physical disease. Thus questions, for example, about shortness of breath, palpitation, sweating and dizziness, are excluded, as although they are prominent somatic symptoms of anxiety they are present in patients with systemic disease, particularly cardiovascular and respiratory conditions. The scale is quick and easy to complete, taking less than ten minutes on most occasions, and has been validated in many studies.

THE TAYLOR MANIFEST ANXIETY SCALE

This scale was extremely popular in the 1950s and 1960s as a measure of anxiety. The original scale (Taylor, 1953) suggested that 50 questions covering the symptoms of anxiety could be an accurate measurement of anxious mood. In fact, the scale, which was developed from the Minnesota Multiphasic Personality Inventory (MMPI), is not really a measure of state anxiety at all but a measure of anxious traits as much as anxious symptoms. Questions such as "I have often felt that

HAD Scale

Name: _____   Date: _____

Doctors are aware that emotions play an important part in most illnesses. If your doctor knows about these feelings he will be able to help you more.

This questionnaire is designed to help your doctor to know how you feel. Read each item and place a firm tick in the box opposite the reply which comes closest to how you have been feeling in the past week.

Don't take too long over your replies: your immediate reaction to each item will probably be more accurate than a long thought-out response.

A D

I feel tense or "would up":
- Most of the time 3
- A lot of the time 2
- Time to time, Occasionally 1
- Not at all 0

I still enjoy the things I used to enjoy:
- Definitely as much 0
- Not quite so much 1
- Only a little 2
- Hardly at all 3

I get a sort of frightened feeling as if something awful is about to happen:
- Very definitely and quite badly 3
- Yes, but not too badly 2
- A little, but it doesn't worry me 1
- Not at all 0

I can laugh and see the funny side of things:
- As much as I always could 0
- Not quite so much now 1
- Definitely not so much now 2
- Not at all 3

Worrying thoughts go through my mind;
- A great deal of the time 3
- A lot of the time 2
- From time to time but not too often . 1
- Only occasionally 0

I feel cheerful:
- Not at all 3
- Not often 2
- Sometimes 1
- Most of the time 0

I can sit at ease and feel relaxed:
- Definitely 0
- Usually 1
- Not often 2
- Not at all 3

A D

I feel as if I am slowed down:
- Nearly all the time 3
- Very often 2
- Sometimes 1
- Not at all 0

I get a sort of frightened feeling like "butterflies" in the stomach:
- Not at all 0
- Occasionally 1
- Quite often 2
- Very often 3

I have lost interest in my appearance:
- Definitely 3
- I dont't take so much care as I should 2
- I may not take quite as much care 1
- I take just as much care as ever 0

I feel restless as if I have to be on the move:
- Very much indeed 3
- Quite a lot 2
- Not very much 1
- Not at all 0

I look forward with enjoyment to things:
- As much as ever I did 0
- Rather less than I used to 1
- Definitely less than I used to 2
- Hardly at all 3

I get sudden feelings of panic:
- Very often indeed 3
- Quite often 2
- Not very often 1
- Not at all 0

I can enjoy a good book or radio or TV programme:
- Often 0
- Sometimes 1
- Not often 2
- Very seldom 3

Fig. 2.3 The Hospital Anxiety and Depression Scale (HADS). The scores for the depression (D) and anxiety (A) sections are totalled separately.

I face so many difficulties I could not overcome them" are clearly not measuring current anxiety and it is most unfortunate that the scale was called a "manifest anxiety" scale. It really belongs to the history of anxiety measurement.

OTHER SELF-RATING SCALES

The Symptom Check List (SCL-90) is a well-established self-rating questionnaire for neurotic symptoms that includes a separate section for anxiety (Derogatis *et al.*, 1974). Panic attacks are not normally rated through the use of rating scales. A common approach is to use the criteria for the diagnosis of panic disorder (see Chapter 5) and list these when assessing patients.

OBSERVER-RATED SCALES

These scales take longer to complete than self-rating scales, but even under these circumstances, rarely take much longer than 15 minutes. Most of them give reliable and consistent records and commonly include an element of observation as well as assessing anxious symptomatology by direct questions to the patient. Although they are technically rigidly conducted interviews in which the questions are asked in a fixed order, in practice it is better to have the flexibility of a semi-structured interview when administering these scales because otherwise the flow of presentation can get distorted.

HAMILTON ANXIETY SCALE

This scale, also called the Hamilton Rating Scale for Anxiety (HSRA) but more commonly abbreviated to HAM-A to distinguish it from the equivalent depression scale (HAM-D), was the first to be introduced to psychiatry through the technique of factor analysis. Although factor analysis had been used by many other, particularly by Cattell in his pioneering work on personality, the 16-PF scale, from which an anxiety scale was developed (Cattell, 1957), Hamilton was the first to use factor analysis for observer ratings of psychiatric patients. The scale (Fig. 2.4) consists of fourteen items originally scored on a five-point scale but some times modified to smaller numbers for some categories. Factor analysis revealed two major factors, one more general factor of anxiety and a second a bipolar factor separating psychological symptoms from somatic symptoms. The scale continues to be used widely but has been somewhat superseded in recent years by greater use of self-rating scales.

CLINICAL ANXIETY SCALE (CAS)

One of the criticisms of the Hamilton anxiety scale is its recording of symptoms such as depression and problems with memory which are not strictly part of anxious symptomatology. However, because they are common in people with anxiety (mainly because of the overlap between anxiety and depression), it is reasonable to argue that they should be included. Snaith and his colleagues (1982) argued that if the items in the Hamilton scale were confined to anxiety, together with its psychological and somatic components, it would be more sensitive. The scale consists of seven items, each scored on a five-point scale (Fig. 2.5); despite the scale having definite merits it has not superseded the Hamilton anxiety scale to any significant extent. This is perhaps unfortunate as it is shorter than the Hamilton anxiety scale and is a purer measure of anxiety.

IRRITABILITY, DEPRESSION AND ANXIETY (IDA) SCALE

This scale (Snaith et al., 1978) is primarily used to assess irritability, which is one of the key elements of anxiety. By combining measures of anxiety and depression, they also succeeded in hiding those elements referring to irritability which tends to have more negative connotations than mood problems. The scale consists of 18 items each scored on a

Patient Name: Date:

0 = Absent
1 = Mild
2 = Moderate
3 = Severe
4 = Very severe, grossly disabling
Answer every question by entering numeral in appropriate box.   Score

ANXIOUS MOOD
Worries, anticipation of the worst, fearful anticipation, irritability

TENSION
Feeling of tension, fatiguability, startle response, moved to tears easily, trembling,
feelings of restlessness, inability to relax

FEARS
Of dark, of strangers, of being left alone, of animals, of traffic, of crowds

INSOMNIA
Difficulty in falling asleep, broken sleep, unsatisfying sleep and fatigue on waking,
dreams, nightmares, night terrors

INTELLECTUAL
Difficulty in concentration, poor memory

DEPRESSED MOOD
Loss of interest, lack of pleasure in hobbies, depression, early waking, diurnal
swing

SOMATIC (Muscular)
Pains and aches, twitchings, stiffness, myoclonic jerks, grinding of teeth, unsteady
voice, increased muscular tone

SOMATIC (Sensory)
Tinnitus, blurring vision, hot and cold flushes, feelings of weakness, pricking
sensation

CARDIOVASCULAR SYMPTOMS
Tachycardia, palpitations, pain in chest, throbbing of vessels, fainting feelings,
sighing, dyspnoea

Fig. 2.4 Hamilton Anxiety Scale.

Score

RESPIRATORY SYMPTOMS
Pressure of constriction in chest, choking feelings, sighing, dyspnoea

GASTROINTESTINAL SYMPTOMS
Difficulty in swallowing, wind, abdominal pain, burning sensations, abdominal fullness,
nausea, vomiting, borborygmi, looseness of bowels, loss of weight, constipation

GENITOURINARY SYMPTOMS
Frequency of micturition, urgency of micturition, amenorrhoea, menorrhagia,
development of frigidity, premature ejaculation, loss of libido, impotence

AUTONOMIC SYMPTOMS
Dry mouth, flushing, pallor, tendency to sweat, giddiness, tension headache, raising
of hair

BEHAVIOUR AT INTERVIEW
Fidgeting, restlessness or pacing, tremor of hands, furrowed brow, strained face,
sighing or rapid respiration, facial pallor, swallowing etc.

TOTAL

Fig. 2.4 (*Continued*)

four-point scale. Eight of these are concerned with irritability (Fig. 2.6).
The scale deserves to be more widely used as irritability is an important
symptom associated with anxiety (and other emotions) that is often
overlooked.

BRIEF ANXIETY SCALE (BAS)

This scale has been developed from the Comprehensive
Psychopathological Rating Scale (CPRS), a scale which records the full
range of psychopathology (Åsberg *et al.*, 1978). The original consists
of 65 items, of which 40 are scored from responses to questions and
25 from observation of the patient. The BAS (Brief Anxiety Scale)

1. Psychic Tension

(care should be taken to distinguish tension from muscular tension–see next item).

Score 4:   Very marked and distressing feeling of being "on edge", "keyed up", "wound up" or "nervous" which persists with little change throughout the waking hours

Score 3:   As above, but with some fluctuation of severity during the course of the day

Score 2:   A definite experience of being tense which is sufficient to cause some, although not severe, distress

Score 1:   A slight feeling of being tense which does not cause distress

Score 0:   No feeling of being tense apart from the normal degree of tension experienced in response to stress and which is acceptable as normal for the population

2. Ability to Relax (muscular tension)

Score 4:   The experience of severe tension throughout much of the bodily musculature which may be accompanied by such symptoms as pain, stiffness, spasmodic contractions, and lack of control over movements. The experience is present throughout most of the waking day and there is no ability to produce relaxation at will

Score 3:   As above, but the muscular tension may only be experienced in certain groups of muscles and may fluctuate in severity throughout the day

Score 2:   A definite experience of muscular tension in some part of the musculature sufficient to cause some, but not severe, distress

Score 1:   Slight recurrent muscular tension of which the patient is aware but which does not cause distress. Very mild degrees of tension headache or pain in other groups of muscles should be scored here

Score 0:   No subjective muscular tension or, if any is experienced, it can easily be controlled at will

3. Startle Response (hyperarousability)

Score 4:   Unexpected noise causes severe distress so that the patient may complain in some such phrase as "I jump out of my skin". Distress is experienced in psychic and somatic modalities so that, in addition to the experience of fright, there is muscular activity and autonomic symptoms such as sweating or palpitation

Fig. 2.5 Clinical Anxiety Scale.

Score 3: Unexpected noise causes severe distress in psychic or somatic, but not in both modalities

Score 2: Unexpected noise causes definite but not severe distress

Score 1: The patient agrees that he is slightly "jumpy" but it not distressed by this

Score 0: The degree of startle response is entirely acceptable as normal for the population

4. Worrying (The assessment must take into account the degree to which worry is out of proportion to actual stress)

Score 4: The patient experiences almost continuous preoccupation with painful thoughts which cannot be stopped voluntarily and the distress is quite out of proportion to the subject matter of thoughts

Score 3: As above, but there is some fluctuation in intensity throughout the waking hours and the distressing thoughts may cease for an hour or two, especially if the patient is distracted by activity requiring his attention

Score 2: Painful thoughts out of proportion to the patients situation keep intruding into consciousness but this does not cause much distress

Score 1: The patient agrees that he tends to worry a little more than necessary about minor matters but this does not cause much distress

Score 0: The tendency to worry is accepted as being normal for the population; for instance even marked worrying over a severe financial crisis or unexpected illness in a relative should be scored as 0 if it is judged to be entirely in keeping with the degree of stress

5. Apprehension

Score 4: The experience is that of being on the brink of some disaster which cannot be explained. The experience need not be continuous and may occur in short bursts several times a day

Score 3: As above, but the experience does not occur more than once a day

Score 2: A sensation of groundless apprehension of disaster which is not severe although it causes definite distress. The patient may not use strong terms such as "disaster" or "catastrophy" but may express his experience in some such phrase as "I feel as if something bad is about to happen"

Fig. 2.5 (*Continued*)

Score 1: A slight degree of apprehensiveness of which the patient is aware but which does not cause distress

Score 0: No experience of groundless anticipation of disaster

6. Restlessness

Score 4: The patient is unable to keep still for more than a few minutes and engages in restless pacing or other purposeless activity

Score 3: As above, but he is able to keep still for an hour or so at a time

Score 2: There is a feeling of "needing to be on the move" which causes some, but not severe, distress

Score 1: Slight experience of restlessness which causes no distress

Score 0: Absense of restlessness

7. Panic attacks

Score 4: Episodes, occurring several times a day, of the sudden experience of groundless terror accompanied by marked automonic symptoms, feelings of imminent collapse or loss of control over reason and self-integrity

Score 3: As above, but the episodes do not occur more than once a day

Score 2: The episodes may occur only once or twice a week; they are generally less severe than described above but still cause distress

Score 1: Episodic slight increases in the level of anxiety which are only precipitated by definite events or activities. For instance, the experience of a patient who is recovering from agoraphobia and who experiences a perceptible rise of anxiety on leaving the house would be scored here

Score 0: No episodic sudden increase in the level of anxiety

Fig. 2.5 (*Continued*)

Clinical Anxiety Scale–Assessment Sheet

Patient Name: Date:

Item	SCORE
1. Psychic tension	
2. Ability to relax	
3. Startle response	
4. Worrying	
5. Apprehension	
6. Restlessness	
7. Panic attacks	
TOTAL SCORE	

Interpretation of Results

Score	Probable Diagnosis
0–4	Normal/Recovered
5–10	Mild anxiety
11–16	Moderate anxiety
17–24	Severe anxiety

Fig. 2.5 (*Continued*)

(Tyrer *et al.*, 1984) consists of ten questions from the CPRS, eight from the subjective symptom section and two from the observation section. The CPRS scale score all the items on a four-point scale, but the BAS (Fig. 2.7) extends this to a seven-point scale to allow for greater sensitivity of scoring.

The BAS is similar to the Montgomery and Åsberg depression rating scale (MADRAS), a ten-point scale also derived from the CPRS, which uses a similar expanded seven-point scale (Montgomery and Åsberg, 1979). Two of the questions in the MADRAS (insomnia and panic) are also included in the BAS and so scores for the two scales are bound to be intercorrelated to some extent. Some overlap is hardly unexpected in view of the common association of depression and anxiety.

Patient Name: Date:

Instructions for use

First write your name and date in the space above. This form has been designed so that you can show how you have been feeling in the past few days.

Read each item in turn and the UNDERLINE the response which best shows how you are feeling or have been feeling in the past few days.

Ignore the letters and numbers at the right-hand side and at the end of the questionnaire.

Make sure you complete all questions.

	Fold here
I feel cheerful:	D
Yes, definitely	0
Yes, sometimes	1
No, not much	2
No, not at all	3

I can sit down and relax quite easily:	A
Yes, definitely	0
Yes, sometimes	1
No, not much	2
No, not at all	3

Fig. 2.6 Irritability, Depression and Anxiety (IDA) Scale.

Fold here

My appetite is:	D
Very poor	3
Fairly poor	2
Quite good	1
Very good	0

I lose my temper and shout or snap at others:	O
Yes, definitely	3
Yes, sometimes	2
No, not much	1
No, not at all	0

I can laugh and feel amused:	D
Yes, definitely	0
Yes, sometimes	1
No, not much	2
No, not at all	3

I feel I might lose control and hit or hurt someone:	O
Sometimes	3
Occasionally	2
Rarely	1
Never	0

I have an uncomfortable feeling like butterflies in the stomach:	A
Yes, definitely	3
Yes, sometimes	2
Not very often	1
Not at all	0

The thought of hurting myself occurs to me:	I
Sometimes	3
Not very often	2
Hardly ever	1
Not at all	0

I'm awake before I need to get up:	D
For 2 hours or more	3
For about 1 hour	2
For less than an hour	1
Not at all, I sleep until it is time to get up	0

Fig. 2.6 (*Continued*)

Fold here

I feel tense or "wound up":   A

    Yes, definitely   3

    Yes, sometimes   2

    No, not much   I

    No, not at all   0

I feel like harming myself: I

    Yes, definitely   3

    Yes, sometimes   2

    No, not much   I

    No, not at all   0

I have kept up my old interests: D

    Yes, most of them   0

    Yes, some of them   I

    No, not many of them   2

    No, none of them   3

I am patient with other people: O

    All the time   0

    Most of the time   I

    Some of the time   2

    Hardly ever   3

I get scared or panicky for no very good reason: A

    Yes, definitely   3

    Yes, sometimes   2

    No, not much   I

    No, not at all   0

I get angry with myself or call myself names: I

    Yes, definitely   3

    Yes, sometimes   2

    Not often   I

    Not at all   0

People upset me so that I feel like slamming doors or banging about: O

    Yes, often   3

    Yes, occasionally   2

    Only occasionally   I

    Not at all   0

Fig. 2.6 (*Continued*)

Fold here

I can go out on my own without feeling anxious:	A
Yes, always	0
Yes, sometimes	I
No, not often	2
No, I never can	3

Lately I have been getting annoyed with myself:	I
Very much so	3
Rather a lot	2
Not much	I
Not at all	0

IDA Scale–Score Interpretation Guide

Depression scores:	total items marked	D	borderline range: 4–6	☐
Anxiety scores:	total items marked	A	borderline range: 6–8	☐
Inward irritability:	total items marked	I	borderline range: 4–6	☐
Outward irritability:	total items marked	O	borderline range: 5–7	☐

Fig. 2.6 (*Continued*)

ASSESSMENTS OF PHOBIC SYMPTOMS

There are many specific scales for recording agoraphobia, social phobia and specific phobias that are described elsewhere (Marks, 1987). The discussion here will be confined to common assessments that can be used for a wide variety of phobias.

FEAR QUESTIONNAIRE

This scale is a brief questionnaire intended for the assessment of change in patients being treated for phobic disorders. It identifies the main phobias of the patient as well as a global phobia rating, and also allows subscores to be developed for agoraphobia and social phobia, together with the common phobia of blood injury (Marks and Mathews, 1979) (Fig. 2.8). This has subsequently been modified to extend its range to all phobias and their avoidance in the Marks-Sheehan Scale (Fig. 2.9).

STRUCTURED INTERVIEW SCHEDULES FOR ASSESSING ANXIETY

There are several diagnostic schedules used to diagnose the different anxiety disorders. However, they are not strictly relevant in measuring

1. Inner Tension
   Representing feelings of ill-defined discomfort, edginess, inner turmoil, mental tension mounting to panic, dread and anguish. Rate according to intensity, frequency, duration and extent of reassurance called for.

   0 Placid. Only fleeting inner tension
   1
   2 Occasional feelings of edginess and ill defined discomfort
   3
   4 Continuous feelings of inner tension, or intermittent which the patient can only master with difficulty
   5
   6 Unrelenting dread or anguish

2. Hostile Feelings
   Representing anger, hostility and aggressive feelings regardless of whether they are acted or not. Rate according to intensity, frequency and the amount of provocation tolerated.

   0 Not easily angered
   1
   2 Easily angered. Reports which are easily dissipated
   3
   4 Reacts to provocation with excessive anger and hostility
   5
   6 Persistent anger, rage or intense hatred which is difficult or impossible to control

Fig. 2.7 The Brief Scale for Anxiety.

3. Hypochondriasis
Representing exaggerated preoccupation or unrealistic worrying about ill health or disease. Distinguish from worrying over trifles and aches and pains.

0   No particular preoccupation with ill health

1

2   Reacting to dysfunction with foreboding. Exaggerated fear of disease

3

4   Convinced that there is some disease but can be reassurred, if only briefly

5

6   Incapacitating or absurd hypochondriacal convictions (body rotting away, bowels have not worked for months)

---

4. Worrying Over Trifles
Representing apprehension and undue concern over trifles which is difficult to stop and out of proportion to the circumstances.

0   No particular worries

1

2   Undue concern, worrying that can be shaken off

3

4   Apprehensive and bothered about the trifles by routines

5

6   Unrelenting and often painful worrying, reassurance is ineffective

---

5. Phobias
Representing feelings of unreasonable fear in specific situation (such as buses, supermarkets, crowds, feeling enclosed)

0   No phobias

1

2   Feeling of discomfort in particular situations which can be mastered without help or by taking simple precautions like avoiding rush hours when possible

3

4   Certain situations consistently provoked marked discomfort and are avoided without impairing social performance

5

6   Incapacitating which severely restrict activities, eg. completely unable to leave home

---

Fig. 2.7 (*Continued*)

6. Reduced Sleep
Representing a subjective experience of reduced duration or depth of sleep compared to the subject's own normal pattern when well.

0 Sleeps as usual
I
2 Slight difficulty dropping off to sleep or slightly reduced light or fitful sleep
3
4 Sleep reduced or broken by at least 2 hours
5
6 Less than two or three hours sleep

---

7. Autonomic Disturbances
Representing descriptions of palpitations, breathing difficulties, dizziness, increased sweating, cold hands and feet, dry mouth, indigestion, diarrhoea, frequent micturition. Distinguish from inner tension and aches and pains.

0 No autonomic disturbances
I
2 Occasional autonomic symptoms which occur under emotional stress
3
4 Frequent or intense autonomic disturbances which are experienced as discomforting or socially inconvenient
5
6 Very frequent autonomic disturbances which interrupt other activities or are incapacitating

---

8. Aches and Pains
Representing reports of bodily discomfort, aches and pains. Rate according to intensity, frequency and duration and also request for relief. Disregard any symptom of organic cause. Distinguish for hypochondriasis, autonomic disturbance, and muscular tension.

0 Absent or transient aches
I
2 Occasional definite aches and pains
3
4 Prolonged and inconvenient aches and pains. Requests for effective analgesics
5
6 Severely interfering or crippling pains

Fig. 2.7 (*Continued*)

9. Autonomic Disturbances

Representing signs of autonomic dysfunction, hyperventilation or frequent sighing, blushing, sweating, cold hands, enlarged pupils and dry mouth, fainting

0 No observed autonomic disturbances

1

2 Occasional or slight autonomic disturbances such as blushing or sweating under stress

3

4 Obvious autonomic disturbance on several occasions even when not under stress

5

6 Autonomic disturbances which disrupt the interview

10. Muscular Tension

Representing observed muscular tension as shown in facial expression, posture and movements.

0 Appears relaxed

1

2 Slightly tense face and posture

3

4 Moderately tense posture and face (easily seen in jaw and neck muscles). Does not seem to find a relaxed position when sitting. Stiff and awkward movements

5

6 Strikingly tense. Often sits hunched and rigidly upright at the edge of the chair

Brief Scale for Anxiety–Assessment Sheet

Patient Name: Date:

Item	SCORE
1. Inner Tension	
2. Hostile Feelings	
3. Hypochondriasis	
4. Worrying over Trifles	

Fig. 2.7 (*Continued*)

SCORE

	SCORE
5. Phobias	
6. Reduced Sleep	
7. Autonomic Disturbances (i)	
8. Aches and Pains	
9. Autonomic Disturbances (ii)	
10. Muscular Tension	
TOTAL SCORE	

Fig . 2.7 (*Continued*)

Patient Name: Date:

Choose a number from the scale below how much you would avoid each of the situations listed below because of fear or other unpleasant feelings. Then write the number you choose in the box opposite each situation.

0 Would not avoid it
1
2 Slightly avoid it
3
4 Definitely avoid it
5
6 Markedly avoid it
7
8 Always avoid it

1. Main phobia you want treated (describe in your own words)

2. Injections or minor surgery

3. Eating or drinking with other people

Fig. 2.8 Fear Questionnaire (Marks and Mathews).

4. Hospitals ☐

5. Travelling alone by bus or coach ☐

6. Walking alone in busy streets ☐

7. Being watched or stared at ☐

8. Going into crowded shops ☐

9. Talking to people in authority ☐

10. Slight of blood ☐

11. Being criticised ☐

12. Going alone far from home ☐

13. Thought of injury or illness ☐

14. Speaking or acting to an audience ☐

15. Large open spaces ☐

16. Going to the dentist ☐

17. Other situations (describe) ☐

leave blank ☐☐☐☐

Now choose a number from the scale below to show how much you are troubled by each problem listed and write the number in the box opposite.

0   Hardly at all
1
2   Slightly troublesome
3
4   Definitely troublesome
5
6   Markedly troublesome
7
8   Very Severely troublesome

Fig. 2.8 (*Continued*)

Score

18. Feeling miserable or depressed ☐

19. Feeling irritable or angry ☐

20. Feeling tense or panicky ☐

21. Upsetting thoughts coming into your mind ☐

22. Feeling you or your surroundings are strange or unreal ☐

23. Other feelings (describe) ☐

TOTAL ☐

How would you rate the present state of your phobic symptoms on the scale below?

0 No phobias present
1
2 Slightly disturbing/not really disabling
3
4 Definitely disturbing/disabling
5
6 Markedly disturbing/disabling
7
8 Very Severely disturbing/disabling

Please circle one number between 0 and 8.

Fig. 2.8 (*Continued*)

anxiety as such but for coding the different symptoms into the current psychiatric classifications. Because of the problems of comorbidity (co-occurrence of several diagnoses) in anxiety disorders (Barlow *et al.*, 1986), it is preferable to use general schedules that include all diagnoses. Examples include The Composite International Diagnostic Interview (Robins *et al.*, 1988), the Structured Interview Schedule for DSM-IV (Spitzer and Williams, 1995), Anxiety Disorders Interview Schedule (ADIS) (Barlow, 1988), and OPCRIT (an interview procedure that allows conversion of the data obtained to more than one diagnostic system (McGuffin *et al.*, 1991).

MAKING REPEATED MEASURES OF ANXIETY

Although it is common for the measure of anxiety to be recorded retrospectively in, for example, clinical trials for new anti-anxiety drugs, it is better to record anxiety prospectively by serial recording at appropriate times. Although this may be an obvious requirement when recording, for example, the anxiety of someone in advance, during and after an activity such as a parachute jump, it is important to realise that anxiety changes dramatically from hour to hour independently of any major events.

The serial recordings of somatic symptoms of anxiety and anxiety as a whole, are shown for one individual in Fig. 2.10. The subject was a patient who had nausea as a prominent feature and it was suspected to be directly related to anxiety, so both the somatic symptom (nausea) and anxiety were recorded simultaneously over a three-week period. The main purpose of the experiment was to assess the relationship between nausea and anxiety as a whole, and a fairly close relationship was identified (the correlation between anxiety and the symptom of nausea was 0.52). However, the figure is shown to illustrate how much anxiety changes during the cause of an average week in the life of someone with pathological anxiety (and may well be similar in those with more normal anxiety).

To fill out the phobia scale below, circle a number between 0 and 10 in the top row of each section to show how much you fear a situation, and a number between 0 and 4 in the bottom row to show how much you avoid that situation. Use the scales below as a guide.

How much do you *fear* the situations named below?

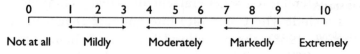

Fig. 2.9 Phobia Scale (Marks and Sheehan).

How much do you *avoid* the situations named below?

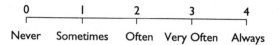

1. Main phobias you want
   treated

   Phobia 1 Specify: Fear   0 1 2 3 4 5 6 7 8 9 10

                         Avoidance   0 1 2 3 4

   Phobia 2 Specify: Fear   0 1 2 3 4 5 6 7 8 9 10

                         Avoidance   0 1 2 3 4

   Phobia 3 Specify: Fear   0 1 2 3 4 5 6 7 8 9 10

                         Avoidance   0 1 2 3 4

   Phobia 4 Specify: Fear   0 1 2 3 4 5 6 7 8 9 10

                         Avoidance   0 1 2 3 4

2. Going far from home alone   Fear   0 1 2 3 4 5 6 7 8 9 10

                         Avoidance   0 1 2 3 4

3. Situations associated with   Fear   0 1 2 3 4 5 6 7 8 9 10
   sudden unexpected attacks   Avoidance   0 1 2 3 4
   of panic/anxiety that occur
   with little or no stress

4. Traveling on buses,   Fear   0 1 2 3 4 5 6 7 8 9 10
   subways, trains, or in cars   Avoidance   0 1 2 3 4

5. Crowded places (e.g.   Fear   0 1 2 3 4 5 6 7 8 9 10
   shopping, sports events,   Avoidance   0 1 2 3 4
   theaters)

6. Large open spaces   Fear   0 1 2 3 4 5 6 7 8 9 10

                         Avoidance   0 1 2 3 4

7. Feeling trapped or caught   Fear   0 1 2 3 4 5 6 7 8 9 10
   in closed spaces   Avoidance   0 1 2 3 4

8. Being left alone   Fear   0 1 2 3 4 5 6 7 8 9 10

                         Avoidance   0 1 2 3 4

Fig. 2.9 (*Continued*)

9. The thought of physical   Fear   0 1 2 3 4 5 6 7 8 9 10
   injury or illness   Avoidance   0 1 2 3 4

10. Hearing or reading about   Fear   0 1 2 3 4 5 6 7 8 9 10
    health topics or disease   Avoidance   0 1 2 3 4

11. Eating, drinking, or writing Fear   0 1 2 3 4 5 6 7 8 9 10
    in public   Avoidance   0 1 2 3 4

12. Being watched or being the   Fear   0 1 2 3 4 5 6 7 8 9 10
    focus of attention   Avoidance   0 1 2 3 4

13. Begin with others because   Fear   0 1 2 3 4 5 6 7 8 9 10
    you are very self-conscious Avoidance 0 1 2 3 4

14. Specify situations other   _____
    than those listed above   _____
    that frighten you: _____

15. Specify farthest distance   _____
    you can go alone: _____

Rate the present state of your phobias overall on the scale below. Circle the number you select.

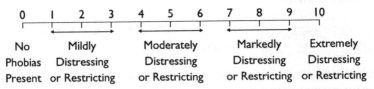

| 0 | 1 | 2 | 3 | 4 | 5 | 6 | 7 | 8 | 9 | 10 |

No   Mildly   Moderately   Markedly   Extremely
Phobias   Distressing   Distressing   Distressing   Distressing
Present   or Restricting   or Restricting   or Restricting   or Restricting

This scale was adapted from the work of I. M. Marks and modified for use in the United States. Those interested in the original work can consult his book *Living with Fear* (see Further Reading).

Fig. 2.9 (*Continued*)

The retrospective assessment of such anxiety is not nearly as easy as it appears. If a subject has been well for nearly the whole of the two-week period but has a serious panic attack the day before the assessment is made, he or she is likely to score highly on a scale for anxiety because the symptoms have been coloured to a great extent by the recent attack.

If, however, the panic was at the beginning of the two-week period and all has gone well since then, the influence of the attack would almost certainly be less and may even be forgotten altogether. Serial prospective recording of anxiety is therefore likely to be more valid than retrospective assessment, and short retrospective ratings (e.g. for periods of one week or less) are likely to be more valid than those involving longer periods between assessments.

AGREEMENT BETWEEN QUESTIONNAIRES AND RATING SCALES FOR ANXIETY

The level of agreement between self-ratings and observer-ratings is generally high. During the Nottingham Study of Neurotic Disorder in which self-ratings using the HADS-A and BAS were recorded serially with scores recorded over the previous two weeks on each occasion, the correlations between the two measures were consistently high on all occasions of testing (Table 2.1).

It is difficult to say whether subject or assessor ratings are more reliable if a decision has to made about a specific choice. It is best not to make a choice if one can be avoided, the main purpose of recording self-ratings and observer-ratings of anxiety being to demonstrate consistency. Thus, for example, if in a trial of two treatments it was found that observer-ratings of anxiety show significant advantage of one treatment over the other, but that no difference of any sort was demonstrated in self-ratings, it would be reasonable to conclude that the difference shown by the observer rating was not to be trusted and possibly was influenced by pre-existing bias on the part of the assessor, particularly if the nature of the two treatments could not be disguised (e.g. psychological treatment compared with a drug one) (Fig. 2.9). There are other occasions where the difference may hide an important clinical matter. For example, in assessing the therapeutic value of a beta-blocking drug, sotalol, some years ago we chose a sequential statistical design (Armitage, 1960). These designs are economical as, unlike other techniques, they record progress sequentially, and when a boundary in the design is crossed, the trial is terminated. If an inner boundary is crossed, no difference has been demonstrated in the

Table 2.1 Persistent high correlations between anxiety and depressive symptoms in 180 patients with generalised anxiety disorder, dysthymic disorder and panic disorder treated over two years (Nottingham Study of Neurotic Disorder)

Comparison of ratings
   obs = observed, slf = self-rating, – d = depression, a = anxiety

Time (Wks)	No. of pts	obsd/ obsa	obsd/ slfd	obsd/ slfa	obsa/ slfd	obsa/ slfa	slfd/ slfa
0	180	48	59	42	40	55	46
2	178	56	71	62	50	70	61
4	178	69	72	60	61	72	67
6	178	79	79	68	67	72	74
10	179	78	79	71	65	72	75
16	178	78	78	69	67	77	75
32	178	76	73	65	67	75	74
52	172	83	75	73	64	75	76
104	161	82	83	73	70	78	77
Weighted mean (after z-transformation)		73.8	75.0	65.5	61.9	72.3	70.4

   Overall correlations (r) ($\times$ 100)

obsd = Montgomery and Åsberg Rating Scale for Depression (MADRAS) (Montgomery and Åsberg, 1979)
obsa = Brief Anxiety Scale (Tyrer *et al.*, 1984)
slfd = Hospital Anxiety and Depression Scale – depression subscore
slfa = Hospital Anxiety and Depression Scale – anxiety subscore

(Reproduced from *Experimental approaches to anxiety and depression* (eds. Elliott, JM, Heal DJ & Marsden CA), p. 14; John Wiley & Sons, 1992 by kind permission of the publishers)

treatment, and if an outer one is crossed, a significant advantage of one treatment over another has been demonstrated, depending on whether it is the upper or lower boundary.

In our study of sotalol, we treated patients with both sotalol and placebo in a balanced cross-over design, so that each patient received the active drug or placebo in a standard order after balancing the order of administration using a Latin square design (insuring that the first treatment is given on the first or second occasion an equal number of times). After both drugs have been received by each patient, a choice was made: (i) by the patient; (ii) by the assessing psychiatrist (myself) about which drug had been more effective, or a decision "no different" if no preference could be made. The results (Fig. 2.10) were interesting. Although all my assessments suggested patients preferred the active drug to placebo, the patients' assessments suggested there was little difference between them, and when the patients' choices crossed an inner boundary, the trial was terminated.

I feel on balance that my assessments were less sound than those of the patients. One of the most marked effects of beta-adrenoceptor blockade shown with sotalol was a reduction in heart rate and other symptoms such as tremor. Although I, as an external observer, might regard these as beneficial, they were not necessarily perceived as advantageous by the patient, particularly if the symptoms were not of any discomfort to the patient. (Indeed one of my patients with anxiety to whom I offered beta-blockade at one stage, refused the offer absolutely saying, "I want to know what's going on in my body when I'm anxious: if you take away these symptoms from me, then I won't be able to monitor my anxiety and I don't know what might happen; I might explode").

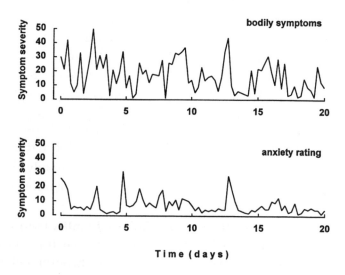

Fig. 2.10 Ratings of bodily symptoms and generalised anxiety completed four times daily in a patient with persistent somatic and anxiety complaints.

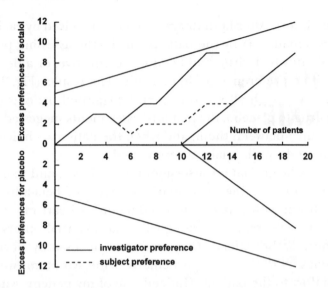

Fig. 2.11 Comparison of investigator (author) and patient preferences in a cross-over trial of sotatol (a beta-blocking drug) and placebo in the treatment of anxiety using a sequential trial design.

What is interesting is that when I presented these results at meetings, I was to some extent criticised by other colleagues for not persisting with trial as the outer boundary (suggesting a significant difference in favour of sotalol) was close to being crossed at the time the trial ended. This was expressed in its strongest form by German colleagues, who may have been too steeped in the traditions of neuropsychiatry in that country when they argued, "Why do you think that the patients' view of the symptoms is better than yours; you are the expert and your view must take priority". We all now tend to be a little more humble in these matters.

SUMMARY

The measurement of anxiety is a relatively simple process in which the most accurate and reliable method is to record the symptoms as soon as possible after they have occurred, either through self-ratings or assessments using a rating scale. All other measures are ancillary and should not be regarded as any substitute for direct mood assessments.

Chapter 3

PSYCHOANALYTICAL CONCEPTS OF ANXIETY

I am not a psychoanalyst and have never been known to have an attraction for this part of psychiatry. However, in a book on anxiety it would be an omission not to discuss at least some aspects of the place of anxiety in psychoanalysis. This is because, quite apart from any intrinsic interest, the nomenclature of anxiety in clinical practice has been influenced greatly by psychoanalysis. The account that follows may offend some with greater knowledge and commitment to psychoanalysis and psychotherapy than my own limited understanding; if so I offer some apology but hope that others may find it more comprehensible than other more advanced texts on the subject.

The history of psychoanalysis is only one hundred years old. From a standing start at the end of the last century, it achieved the distinction of being the predominant influence in psychiatry by the early 1930s, but since then it has been in slow decline. Anxiety was in at the beginning of the rise and a major feature at its time of decline. The importance of anxiety is illustrated by the early heady days of psychoanalysis. Sigmund Freud had returned from hearing Jean Marie Charcot demonstrating his famous patients with "la grande hysterie", most of whom were women, who adopted strange behaviour and dramatic postures that impressed the medical students at the Saltpetrière Hospital in Paris, but gave little indication of the cause and treatment of these conditions.

Charcot taught that these conditions had a neurological basis; Freud guessed the problems lay in the psyche. He returned to Vienna and, during the course of his neurological work with his colleague, Breuer, he came across other patients who showed their hysteria in less dramatic ways than Charcot's patients but had seemed to have a psychological cause for their condition. When Freud looked through the convoluted tunnels of possible explanations for his patients' conditions, he always seemed to finish up in the tunnel marked "sex". To be more specific, the direction over the tunnel read "sexual anxiety". Although many have criticised Freud for this apparent preoccupation with sex throughout his career, there is little doubt that in middle-class Vienna at the turn of the century, there was a neurotic and abnormal preoccupation with never mentioning the subject except in code. It was, therefore, highly likely that many of Freud's patients were in fact preoccupied with this subject whether or not it was the cause of their symptoms. This led to the simple view that a large part of anxiety neurosis was determined by distorted sexual drive (or libido) which was transferred to symptomatic expression when it could not be displayed in other ways.

The fundamental core of psychoanalysis was the concept of the unconscious, the iceberg of the human psyche concealed below the water line of consciousness, with only a small fraction exposed to open view and rational discussion. Psychoanalysis set itself the task of exploring the topography of this hidden mass in the hope of understanding psychopathology in all its forms, from the normal variation of ordinary social intercourse to the most severe of mental illnesses.

Anxiety was at the water-line of the iceberg. If it was understandable and related to clear and unequivocal external causes, it was an acceptable emotion remaining in the exposed part of the iceberg; but if the anxiety was vague and threatening in a way that was pregnant with uncertainty, it was manifest in the submerged part of the iceberg. The psychoanalyst was therefore faced with a difficult dilemma when assessing someone who has manifestations of anxiety; was this a normal, healthy, uncomplicated anxiety unworthy of close enquiry, or was it the distorted anxiety of psychiatric morbidity which had to be dissected and probed before its meaning was understood? When the subsequent development of psychoanalysis made the correct interpretation of this distorted anxiety a main feature, its correct identification at the outset became even more important. In Fig. 3.1, the positions of respectable and unacceptable anxiety are illustrated in a relationship to the iceberg of consciousness.

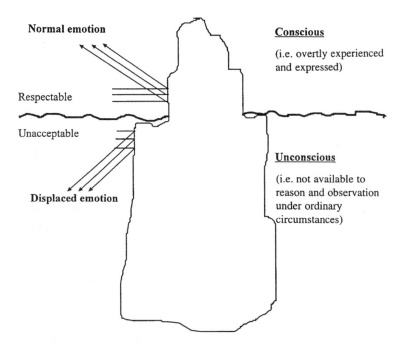

Fig. 3.1 Anxiety and the iceberg of consciousness.

Unacceptable distorted anxiety covered a wide range of possible explanations but central to them are the mental mechanisms of denial and repression. Denial is the ability of the psyche to reject obvious explanations of events because they are too threatening. As a consequence complicated mechanisms are set in operation to cover up what has been denied. These mechanisms can get very complicated indeed. One of the best films to represent the consequences of denial was *The Three Faces of Eve*, a story based on the life of a young woman who aroused intense interest in psychiatry. Eve (the title role was played by Joanna Woodwood in a remarkable performance) was very close to her grandmother and could not accept her loss when she died. As an attempt to overcome this awful event she developed three separate personalities, each very different from the other and manifest at different times. The memory of her grandmother's death was repressed, as indeed were the memories of each of the individual personalities when they changed from one to another, so that Eve's life became a series of individual episodes that were to all intents and purposes unconnected. The outcome of this distortion of anxiety, now called multiple personality disorder, is a rare but important consequence of gross denial and repression.

According to psychoanalytical theory, the reason for denial and repression lie in the operation of the three components of the psyche, the ego, the superego and id. These are now extremely well known concepts and have been caricatured in many ways (e.g. the psychoanalyst is often described "the odd in pursuit of the id") but it is still worth while summarising the three elements.

The ego is the accessible and exposed part of the psyche, equivalent to the conscious element of the iceberg in Fig. 3.1. It is influenced greatly by social conventions, wishes, underlying personality and attitude, and appropriate channelling of basic drives and impulses. It is moulded by experience but constantly influenced by the superego and id. The superego is the moral conscience of the ego, constantly checking that it is behaving appropriately and monitoring its responses. The ego must always fit in with society's expectations and yet still be at ease with itself, a combination of *saviour faire* and *joie de vivre*. The id is the converse of the superego. It represents the basic human drives in their unexpurgated form: lust, greed, sloth, hate and pursuit of pleasure. These drives cannot be allowed free expression in civilised society but they can never be suppressed. The ego represents the acceptable balance between the naked selfish desires of the id and the strictures of the superego, which, like a Victorian governess, attempts to suppress all basic emotions and make them subservient to the higher aims of endeavour, thrift, betterment and altruism, all of which run directly counter to the aims of the id.

It is therefore not surprising that the ego, squeezed on either side by two powerful figures, has to be flexible and accommodating to remain at least partly independent, and this can be done only by diverting the pressures of the id in particular to other parts of the psyche, notably the unconscious. The mechanism of denial — refusing to accept something because it is disturbing to the integrity of the ego — and repression — burying uncomfortable thoughts and emotions that are not acceptable — are intrinsic to ego function. The problem with anxiety is that it can be present in three different forms at different stages of the process: (i) an early stage in which the signal is recognised as posing stress; (ii) at the time it is being processed to a form acceptable to the ego; and (iii) in the last stage as a representation of the conflict in its literal sense, a new presentation of the threatened feeling in a form that can be accommodated within ego function.

Anxiety in any form is therefore judged to be an acceptable emotion and this makes it popular with the ego. Most other emotions are considered less acceptable and may therefore be "converted" into anxiety to allow their expression in disguised form.

The problem for any independent assessment of such anxiety is to determine in which mode the anxiety is functioning and this is a very tall order. Psychoanalytical theory has made it more complicated by postulating another concept, regression. This states that at times of unresolved conflicts, the ego regresses to more primitive levels and any problems are expressed in a form appropriate to that level. This is illustrated in Fig. 3.2, where the ego, represented by a sphere, becomes smaller when regressed and falls down a "developmental funnel" until it is held up by an appropriate obstruction.

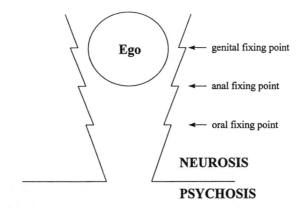

Fig. 3.2 The phenomenon of regression. The ego is represented as a sphere which expresses in symptoms when regressed at different levels. When severely regressed and damaged, it falls through the funnel and becomes expressed at the psychotic level.

The genital, anal and oral phases of developmental repression in Freudian theory (Freud, 1908) are the main obstacles holding up the fall of the ego. The form of expression of anxiety varies from sexual anxiety at the upper level (e.g. frigidity, impotence) to obsessional anxiety characterised by the anxiety of doubt at the intermediate level, and the anxiety of hysteria (oral anxiety) at the lower level. If the damage to the ego becomes too great, it falls through the bottom of the developmental funnel and then becomes psychotic anxiety, anxiety which has no anchor points on which to hold and which is inchoate and terrifying.

Freud and his fellow psychoanalysts were preoccupied with anxiety as a symptom of sexual conflict. In the classical accounts of such anxiety, the hydrodynamic notion of libido (sexual drive) being forced to express itself in one way or another, dominated thinking. For example, agoraphobia, or fear of open spaces, crowded streets and public transport, was reformulated in psychoanalytical thinking as "anxiety hysteria" and became accepted as a formal psychiatric diagnosis. This disorder, predominant in females, was postulated to be caused by fear of the sexual act, a classical conflict between the superego and the id in which, on this particular occasion, the superego had won the battle and was calling the shots. The fear could not be expressed openly (i.e. was denied and repressed) and so the conflict (which could not be denied) had to find ways of expressing itself "in code" as it were, giving a covert message to consciousness that all was not well but in a form that could be regarded as neutral. Thus activities such as crossing roads and travelling through market places, which under ordinary circumstances would arouse no concern, could be explained as symbolic of sexual intercourse if they were presented in certain forms. One way in which these feelings could be squeezed out of the unconscious and passed upwards to consciousness was through the expression of dreams. It was only in this twilight medium (the part of the iceberg at which the water is lapping in Fig. 3.1) that links could be constructed between the conscious and the unconscious. This powerful insight helps to explain why analysis of dreams — Freud's "royal road to the unconscious" — was so important in the psychoanalyst's repertoire.

Although in retrospect this interpretation seems somewhat laughable — if this really was the explanation of agoraphobia, it would be difficult to explain why, for example, it is so common in elderly people and why its persistent prevalence has been maintained despite sexual habits becoming more liberal — the separation of anxiety into neurotic and normal anxiety was a valiant attempt to make sense of neurotic symptomatology while allowing that it appears on the surface to be the same as normal anxiety. This explanation was also an antidote to the tendency, particularly prevalent in the German literature, to define and redefine the symptomatology of psychiatry without understanding its underlying meaning.

It also leads to two other important concepts, those of symptom *conversion* and *substitution*. If an anxiety symptom was treated in isolation, or removed by some treatment specific only to that symptom, it might be suppressed but would not be eliminated unless its cause was also removed. Thus, to take an example from one of Freud's important cases, a young woman presenting with *globus hystericus*, the feeling of being unable to swallow, could have the problem treated directly as a wallowing problem only, which might lead to resolution. However, if the sexual anxiety is postulated as its cause, ambivalence to oral sex, was not addressed by the psychoanalyst, the symptom could be presented in a different form and be converted to vocal paralysis or psychogenic vomiting.

Although psychoanalysts wrestle with anxiety in its various forms, it was never able to give a satisfactory explanation that covered all its ramifications. As there was no means to identify *anxiety-as-a-symptom* from *anxiety-as-a-defence*, it was convenient to slot in any explanation that fitted psychoanalytical theory in general and the specifics of an individual case in particular. It was this catch-all explanation that led to psychoanalytical theory being regarded by many as fanciful, scorned as "*Tales from the Vienna Woods*". Thus, a poor patient, handicapped by anxiety that he or she could not understand, was hardly reassured by a course of treatment that enabled no explanation to be given of such suffering, on the basis that the anxiety experienced may be similar in degree, but now that was known and understandable, it should somehow hurt less.

1895   Transferred libido theory

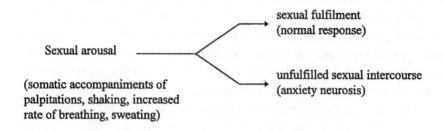

1926   Ego threat theory

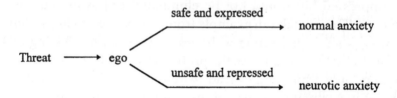

Fig. 3.3 Freud's changing views on the cause of anxiety.

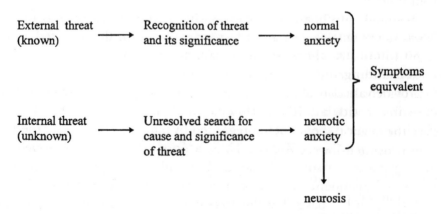

Fig. 3.4 Freud's views on the place of anxiety in the explanation of neurotic disorder.

Later in the course of psychoanalysis, Freud realised that his original explanation of anxiety as displaced libidinal drive must be wrong (Fig. 3.3) and replaced it with a less fundamental hypothesis that neurotic anxiety was created when there was a threat to the ego, whereas normal anxiety could be expressed when there was no threat. He still recognised that anxiety was a fundamental symptom in psychiatric practice and indeed remarked that it was at "the heart of psychoanalysis". Rather than propose an explanation for neurotic anxiety, he confined himself to suggesting that it was "anxiety about a danger that had yet to become known" (Fig. 3.4), thus conceding that psychoanalysis, despite all its attempts, had not yet been able to provide this knowledge. This was perhaps the most modest of all Freud's theories but maybe the most valuable. It explained why pathological anxiety was so much more distressing to the sufferer than normal anxiety; it could not be identified and therefore became much more threatening. Half the solution to the problem of anxiety is in proper recognition of its origin. Just as the patient with delusional mood in schizophrenia suddenly feels better when his mental perturbations crystallise into the primary delusion — "now I realise why so many people are wearing sunglasses; they are all Martians communicating with me by telepathy" — the person with pathological anxiety feels better when recognition dawns and the cause of all the symptoms is displayed. Whether psychoanalysis has helped to provide a good treatment for anxiety disorders is debatable, but it has certainly helped to understand why it underpins so much of mental pathology.

So where has psychoanalysis left psychiatry? What is its legacy to understanding the morbid and health components and is it going to provide valuable new insights in the future? Perhaps it is best to leave the subject with a series of questions that psychoanalysis has posed over the years (usually without receiving a satisfactory answer) rather than provide its own explanations to them:

(i)   When does anxiety cease to have practical value and become a handicap?

(ii)   If anxiety is mainly a symptom indicating other disorder, why is it classified as a disease or a disorder in its own right?

(iii) If anxiety is fundamental to psychopathology, why is it always relegated to the lowest level of the hierarchy of classification?

(iv) If anxiety is a response to threat, what prevents the threat from being perceived?

(v) If anxiety creates a condition with both psychological and bodily consequences in approximately equal degree, why is it that some people present almost entirely with bodily symptoms, others with psychological symptoms only, while others with equal presentation?

(vi) Why do the symptoms of anxiety keep changing if they are indicative of the same fundamental disorder?

(vii) Why are we more anxious when we are vulnerable?

(viii) If conditions such as obsessive-compulsive disorder, post-traumatic stress disorder, generalised anxiety disorder, and somatisation disorder all have anxiety at their core, why is it necessary to provide specific treatments for them; are they not the same disorder?

(ix) If anxiety is a psychiatric disorder like any other psychiatric disorders, why does its treatment almost always lead to dependence? (This criticism is often made of psychoanalysis; the person who only remains well whilst seeing the analyst is said to have a "transference cure" as good health is only maintained by the positive transference (i.e. love) between therapist and client. It is curious that this criticism is not made of drug treatment in quite the same withering way.)

(x) If anxiety is a relatively lowly member of the family of psychiatric disorders, why should it be so difficult to treat and so persistent in its manifestations?

(xi) If anxiety is caused by uncertainty in our lives, why in this age of greater knowledge and understanding of psychological health and disease should it be so prevalent as it was a hundred years ago?

Chapter 4

PHYSIOLOGY OF ANXIETY

All psychological events are reflected in physiological changes in some way but anxiety is by far the best example. Whereas the physiological representation of a wide range of other psychological states has only been identified recently through the new techniques of neuroimaging, the changes in anxiety have been known for centuries and are as old as the history of language itself. Like a refracting lens, the experience of anxiety magnifies a normal physiological function which is usually manifest externally to a relatively untrained observer. This is why anxiety is almost the simplest mood to identify; a highly anxious person shows by expression, appearance and behaviour all the features of the emotion. If the words "I am anxious" were emblazoned over their heads in bright light, it would convey little additional information. All these changes are present on the surface and can be recorded by an observer, often at some distance, so it is not surprising there are internal changes that can be recorded relatively easily.

BODILY CHANGES

"The feeling of anxiety may have linked to it a disturbance of one or more of the bodily functions — such as respiration, heart action, vasomotor innervation or glandular activity. From this combination the patient picks out in particular now one, now another, factor. The proportion in which these elements are mixed in an anxiety attack (Angstzustand) varies to a remarkable degree, and almost every accompanying symptom alone can constitute an attack just as well as can the anxiety itself" (Freud, 1895)

Each one of the external manifestations of anxiety described in the above passage has its own understandable and measurable physiological accompaniment. When people sometimes object to the mental sciences as "black box science", that people measure only the input and output of complex systems and have no idea what is going on in between, they conveniently ignore anxiety. In an individual patient the changes are crystal clear and illustrate why physiologists are more confident in their measurement of anxiety than any other emotion.

THE RACING HEART

The measurement of heart-rate is probably the oldest physiological measurement in medicine. In addition to the sensation of one's own heartbeat at times of anxiety (often expressed as "palpitations"), there are many other ways of measuring heart-rate, the most common of which is the measurement of the pulse, usually by palpation of the radial artery as it comes to the surface just before it enters the hand. Because this measurement is almost the only window into the activities of the inner body, it was given excessive respect by early physicians. Thus the physician, Sir George Baker, attending King George III in the 1788 during his psychiatric disturbance, was forced to infer much from examination of the pulse rate and regularly recorded it almost as an obsession or a talisman that might disclose the key to successful diagnosis. Thus he noticed that "during the extreme severity of pain" the pulse rate fell by one third; that despite being "in a room much heated with company, fires and candles, the pulse was only at 84"; that the pulse was 88 when King George "talked much and with great eagerness and anxiety on things respecting his health", whereas on many other occasions when "the pulse was much quickened" the strokes could not be numbered because of lack of cooperation from the agitated King (Macalpine and Hunter, 1969). In fact, the value of the pulse rate is fairly limited but has the big advantage of being easily measured. Paper records of the pulse are made in the electrocardiogram (ECG) or by a wide range of monitoring equipment. This will record not only the pulse rate but also the inter-beat interval — another related phenomena. However, because these are largely related to activities other than anxious mood, e.g. sinus arrhythmia — increase and decrease in heart-rate accompanying breathing, which itself determines the rate at which blood flows into the heart, the changes that go on in the short-term are of relatively little importance to the emotional state.

A universal finding is that pulse rate is increased in anxiety but, because there is wider inter-individual variation in pulse-rate, it cannot be assumed that a pulse rate of, say, 90 per minute, indicates that individual is anxious. However, if a person has a pulse rate of 90 per minute in a doctor's surgery and one of 70 per minute at rest at home, it is likely that the difference could be accounted for by anxiety only. There are, however, many other reasons for having a high resting pulse rate, including constitutional differences between people, metabolic diseases such as thyrotoxicosis, recent exercise, recent consumption of a heavy meal, and adverse effects of certain drugs. Anxiety can normally be identified as a cause of the rapid heart-rate by means of measuring the pulse when the person is feeling less or more anxious.

Of course, some people complain of anxiety throughout their waking lives, and in such people the evidence that anxiety is the cause of their high pulse rate is only obtained by measuring the pulse during sleep. This is a classical way of separating the high pulse rate of a disorder such as thyrotoxicosis from anxiety; in the thyrotoxic patient the sleeping pulse rate will be equally high. It is also important to appreciate that all states of high emotion, commonly known as high arousal, will have similar effects in raising the pulse rate and so anxiety cannot be assumed. To add further confusion, the vagus nerve, which innervates the heart and reduces its rate when stimulated, can be activated by states of terror, the most severe form of anxiety, and thereby reduces the heart rate. "My heart stopped", is an expression commonly used when people are terrified and indicates that vagal stimulation is in full operation. Having "palpitations", or the feeling of your heart beating in your chest more obviously than usual, may be a consequence of increased heart rate or severely reduced heart rate; it is the latter that produces the more powerful feelings. This is because each heart beat has a job to do, to pump blood round the body, and if the frequency of beat is reduced each beat has to do more. The most powerful contractions of the heart are during intense physical activity (when both rate and power are increased) and during vagal stimulation (when rate is slow and power is great).

THE HEAVING CHEST

When people are anxious they breathe more quickly. They do not breathe more quickly because they need to, as for example happens after a vigorous exercise, but because they are anticipating a quick getaway from the situation that has made them anxious. Unfortunately, as so often happens in modern life, the situation that makes you anxious is often not identified or, if it is, it is not always easy to make an escape without behaviour that may create even more anxiety.

This increased rate of respiration is extremely easy to measure and could be done by simple observation. However, for automatic recording of the respiratory rate, it is common to use devices such as a thermistor, which is taped just in front of the nose, and which responds to temperature changes. When a person breathes in, the air passing the thermistor is cold, but when he breathes out, the air has been warmed by the lungs and the thermistor responds differently. The temperature change is converted into an electrical impulse that can be recorded on a stylus or other forms of recorder (including the measurement of the temperature itself). We therefore get a series of waves, rather like sine waves, with each cycle of respiration (Fig. 4.1).

Because the increased respiratory rate in anxiety is not physiologically justified (i.e. it is not determined by the need to get more oxygen into the lungs), the depth of respiration becomes less than normal. This is illustrated by another method that can be used to record respiratory rate, plethysmography, in which a rubber band around the chest records the expansion and contraction of the chest and therefore also records the changes in the volume of air going in and out of the lungs.

Sometimes the increased rate of respiration is not compensated for adequately by the decreased depth of breathing and too much air comes into the lungs. This is not a problem in itself, since extra oxygen in the

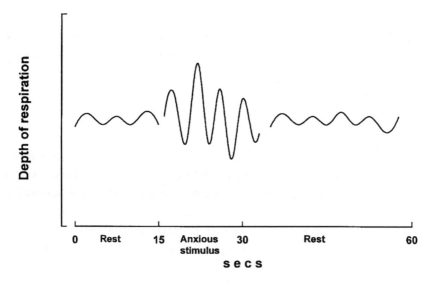

Fig. 4.1 Recording of respiratory rate using a thermistor in a volunteer subject exposed to anxiety (snake in test room).

lungs does no harm, but can create a problem because too much carbon dioxide is evacuated from the lungs by the frequent (over) breathing. Reduced carbon dioxide (hypocapnia) can lead to changes in the acidity of the blood and alter the balance between ionised and unionised calcium. If the proportion of unionised calcium rises, the individual can develop tinglings in the hands and feet which may progress to tetany. This interesting physiological fact, first identified by J B S Haldane, can easily be induced by rapidly over-breathing for several minutes. With low ionised calcium, the nerve conduction becomes disturbed and thus lowers the threshold for nervous impulses to pass to the muscles. Because of this, muscles are induced to contract inappropriately, creating spasm, and these are known as in Trousseau's and Chvostek's signs (spasm of the hand and twitching of the face).

These changes are rapidly reversed by increasing the amount of carbon dioxide in the lungs again, and the reversal can be most conveniently achieved by rebreathing in expired air from the lungs, as for example by putting a paper bag over your mouth and rebreathing a large part of the expired air which contains a higher proportion of carbon dioxide. This well-documented series of physiological events is often misinterpreted by anxious patients and leads to greater anxiety because of the alarm it creates.

THE FURROWED BROW

No cartoonist forgets the furrowed brow in anxiety; the face is such an excellent beacon of our emotional expression. Other muscles in the body are also tense but the brow shows most clearly. The furrows are caused by the scalp muscles contracting excessively and making themselves prominent on the surface because, unlike other parts of the body, the tense muscles cannot expand downwards into the tissues since they are directly placed over the skull. There is little point in this physiological change; these muscles do not become more efficient when they are contracted but they are extremely useful in conveying the emotions of fear and anxiety.

The activity in these muscles can easily be measured by using the electromyogram (EMG). This is a relatively simple procedure involving the placing of electrodes over the relevant muscles and recording the electrical potentials as muscle activity changes. An example of the records in anxiety and at rest is illustrated (Fig. 4.2). Further analyses of the electrical activity can be done by dividing this into different wavebands (spectral analysis) and only the higher frequencies of activity regarded as indices of true muscle activity. Thus the raw ratings shown in Fig. 4.1 can be converted into proportions of voltage in different wavebands (Fig. 4.7). The muscle groups concerned with the furrowed brow together constitute the frontalis muscle and two electrodes placed over the forehead are commonly used with the EMG. However, muscle activity can be recorded in other parts of the body equally easily where muscles are immediately beneath the skin.

Because voluntary muscles, unlike many of the other physiological changes in anxiety, are subject to conscious control, they can be influenced fairly easily by the subject. This is made use of in the technique called biofeedback, which is discussed later.

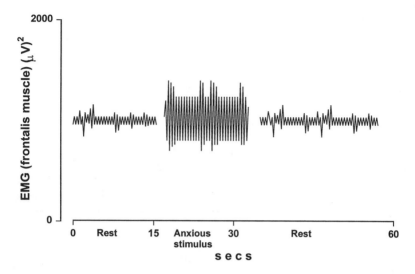

Fig. 4.2 Recording of the electromyogram from the frontalis (forehead) muscle during rest and anxiety in a volunteer subject.

SWEATY PALMS

Although the secretion of sweat is paradoxically controlled by the parasympathetic nervous system (i.e. its autonomic innervation is cholinergic, not adrenergic), it is as much a part of the emergency system of anxiety as the other symptoms described above. Anxious people sweat independently of the need to control their temperature needs (although it is important to acknowledge in this context that hot weather and high humidity will increase sweating quite independently of anxiety), and the changes that take place can easily be measured by electrical changes. The resistance of the skin becomes less when sweating occurs — a salty solution is an excellent conductor of electricity — and this can be measured by direct monitoring of the changes in resistance or in its reciprocal measure, skin conductance. The psychogalvanic reflex (PGR) and galvanic skin response (GSR) record the changes in resistance in response to a stimulus, while skin conductance and spontaneous fluctuations in conductance and resistance are better measures of baseline sweating and, by implication, of anxiety.

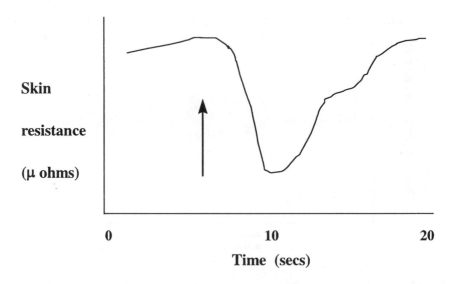

Fig. 4.3 The psychogalvanic reflex (PGR) occuring in response to an anxious stimulus. Note the rapid reduction in resistance followed by a slow return to previous resistance levels.

An example of common changes in skin resistance is shown in Fig. 4.3. An electrical system is set up with voltage being recorded across an area of the skin linked to emotional sweating, usually the thumb and forearm. The decrease in resistance follows the presentation of a click to which the subject has to respond by pressing a button. This is associated with an increase in emotional sweating; the resistance falls suddenly and then recovers quickly to its former level within a few seconds.

The GSR is a useful measure but is not very specific. In addition to responding to changes in temperature and other emotions apart from anxiety, it is very unstable. The common use of skin resistance changes as a lie detector is also subject to a great deal of interpretation. The common way of testing whether the subject is telling a lie, is to repeat a series of neutral words while measuring skin resistance and interposing an emotionally laden word in the sequence. Thus, a subject who claims not to know the first name of a victim he has attacked, could have the name repeated among a sequence of other names. A much greater GSR when this name is mentioned indicates it has special significance even if it is denied openly. Unfortunately, the people who often carry out criminal acts have smaller GSRs than other individuals and, in general, are less anxious.

Although people with anxiety disorders generally have higher skin conductance and greater GSRs than normal individuals and those with non-anxious diagnoses (Gilberstadt and Maley, 1965; Lader and Wing, 1966; Lader, 1967), the individual resistance and conductance levels are usually of less value than the other measures such as the rate of habituation of skin conductance responses (i.e. the rate at which the response diminishes with repeated presentation of the stimulus) (Lader and Wing, 1966).

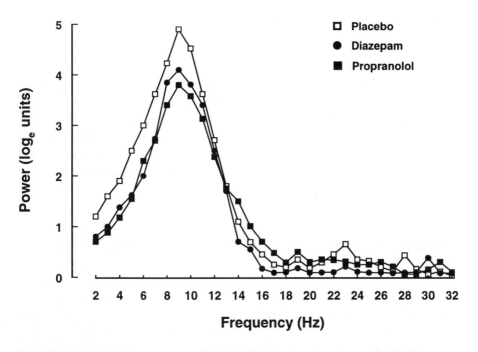

Fig. 4.4 Example of the tremor profiles of 12 anxious patients treated with diazepam (mean 9.6 mg/day), propranolol (120 mg/day) and placebo for one week each in a cross-over trial. There was a significant reduction in tremor with both active drugs at frequencies between 4 and 10 Hz inclusive. *From Tyrer (1976) by permission of Oxford University Press.*

THE SHAKING HAND

Tremor is also a clear physiological accompaniment of anxiety. Such tremor is a quantitative accentuation of physiological tremor, which is predominantly at a frequency of 10 cycles a second (10 Hz), and which, interestingly, is at the same frequency as the alpha rhythm of the electroencephalogram. This is at a higher frequency than the 4–5 Hz frequency of Parkinsonian tremor and has the same profile as normal anxiety (Tyrer and Lader, 1974). When anxious tremor is treated, it decreases in amplitude but not in frequency (Fig. 4.4). Interestingly, the profile of tremor in an individual is like a fingerprint; it is genetically determined, so monozygotic twins have tremor patterns that are much closer than those of dizygous twins (Tyrer and Kasriel, 1975).

BLOOD FLOW

There are also changes in blood flow to the peripheral musculature during anxiety (Kelly and Walter, 1968), with an increase in forearm (muscle) blood flow and a reduction in skin blood flow. The increase in forearm blood flow is highest in anxiety and least in the primary depersonalisation syndrome, an extremely rare condition in which the sufferer is not aroused by any stimulus and stays in a permanent state of unreality.

OTHER PHYSIOLOGICAL CHANGES IN THE BRAIN DURING ANXIETY

Relating evidence from the newer technologies of imaging and cerebral blood flow measurement to symptoms and psychological experiences, is an extremely difficult task and we have only made a short journey down the road of interpreting the mass of data that is currently being collected.

However, the following information is highly relevant to the subject and remains to be further investigated to ensure that there are no artefacts in the data that are leading to false conclusions.

Reiman and his colleagues (1985) have performed a series of investigations of cerebral blood flow in patients with panic disorder and normal controls. They showed a significant asymmetry in the cerebral blood flow of those with panic disorder compared with controls and this asymmetry was particularly marked in the inferior frontal gyrus, a structure that is close to the hippocampus and traditionally part of the limbic system. Such asymmetry in blood flow is likely to be of special significance but it is fair to say that at present this cannot be defined or confirmed precisely.

AUDITORY EVOKED POTENTIALS

Brain activity is difficult to interpret from measures such as the electroencephalogram (EEG) as there are a large number of electrical impulses being generated in the brain at any one time and interpreting these at the surface is often extremely difficult. However, if a particular event can be linked in time to electrical activity, it is possible to identify it against the background of generalised electrical activity by using the technique of averaging (Dawson, 1951).

One of the common events used in experiments is a repeated presentation of a sound and to record brain activity immediately before and after the sound is administered. Subsequently, the data are averaged over all the occasions that the sound has been presented and, because the effects that are independent of the sound being administered tend to be lost in the averaging process, the specific changes associated with hearing the noise become magnified to a marked degree (Fig. 4.5).

The averaged auditory evoked response, commonly abbreviated to AER, is a characteristic response pattern (Fig. 4.5). In normal individuals who are alert and concentrating on hearing the sound, it is a response of reasonable amplitude that is easy to identify. However, in anxious subjects that amplitude of the AER is increased and the latencies before each peak and trough are both reduced. Treatment of anxiety with sedative drugs reduces the amplitude and increases the latency of all components of the evoked response.

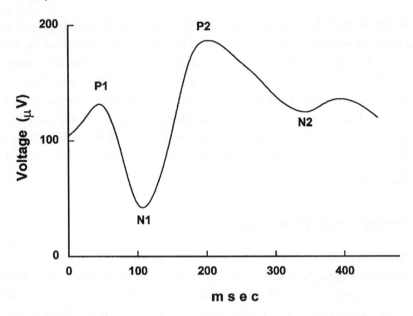

Fig. 4.5 A typical average evoked response (average of 32 EEG records) immediately after hearing a series of auditory clicks.

BASELINE CHANGES IN THE EEG

Although standard EEG consists of a large number of brain waves of different frequencies that make no apparent sense, when the recordings are subjected to a procedure known as spectral analysis, whereby the frequencies of different wave patterns can be banded, some interesting patterns can be identified. When the eyes are open the characteristic frequency of activity is a fast one of around 25–40 cycles (Hz) (β- or beta rhythm). With the eyes closed, the predominant rhythm is at a lower level of around 8–13 Hz, characteristically known as the alpha rhythm. In states of drowsiness and sleep and also in young children, there are also a large number of waves of slower frequencies, particularly theta activity at 4–6 Hz and delta activity between 1–4 Hz.

In anxiety an almost universal finding is that the proportion of beta activity is greater, so there is a corresponding reduction of other frequencies and this applies when both the eyes are open or closed.

RELATIONSHIP BETWEEN BODILY SYMPTOMS OF ANXIETY AND PHYSIOLOGICAL CHANGES

It might be expected that there would be a close relationship between the bodily and physiological changes in anxiety. There is, but it is not as clear as one might predict. Our nervous systems are very economical in their handling of incoming stimuli from different parts of the body. "If it changes, take note; if it stays the same, ignore it", is a useful motto for a system under overload. The alternative would mean that our consciousness would be overwhelmed by a mass of stimuli that would prevent adequate notice being taken of really important changes. However, when people become anxious, they get more severe symptoms than they would ever do under normal circumstances, so it would be expected that symptoms would be directly related to the underlying physiological changes.

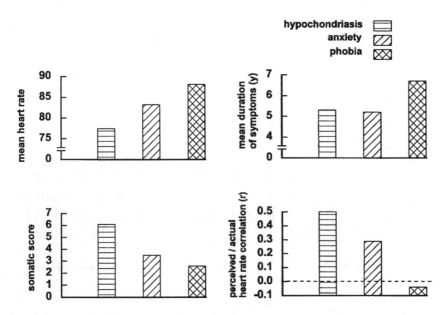

Fig. 4.6 Comparison of mean heart rate, duration of symptoms, somatic score and level of correlation between actual and perceived heart rate in patients with a primary hypochondriacal syndrome (n = 18), anxiety neurosis (n = 23) and phobias (agoraphobia and social phobia) (n = 19).

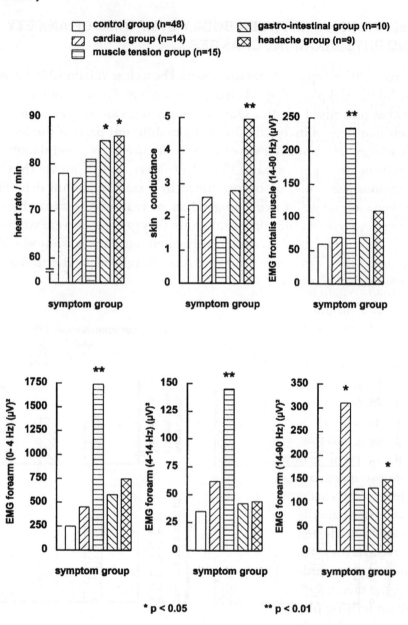

Fig. 4.7 Comparison of physiological activity measured by heart rate, skin conductance and electromyogram (forearm and frontalis muscles) in 48 control subjects and 48 anxious patients separated into four groups on the basis of their main symptoms.

The research findings suggest that when patients are hypochondriacally anxious, they are much more aware of their physiological function than when they have other forms of anxiety. This is illustrated in Fig. 4.6 in which the correlations between the heart rates and perceived heart rates (measured on a 100 mm analog scale) (see Chapter 2) were calculated in 60 anxious patients. These comprised 18 hypochondriacal patients, 19 phobic patients and 23 with generalised anxiety. The heart rates and perceived heart rates were measured during the screening of two short cine-film sequences, one anxiety-reducing and the other tranquillising, so a range of heart rates and anxious feelings were recorded. Despite the fact that the hypochondriacal patients had lower pulse rates than the anxious ones, overall they were significantly more effective in identifying their heart rates successfully (Tyrer *et al.*, 1980).

Anxious patients tend to have a tendency to demonstrate one or more physical symptoms at the expense of others. This was noted many years ago and given the title of "autonomic response specificity" by Lacey and his colleagues (1953). In another study, including some of the patients shown in Fig. 4.6, we compared the physiological measures of heart rate (ECG), forehead (frontalis muscle) and forearm muscle activity (EMG), and sweating (skin conductance) in 48 control subjects and 48 anxious subjects. The anxious patients were classified in terms of their major symptoms into four groups (cardiac, muscular tension, gastrointestinal and headache groups). There was some evidence of "physiological response specificity", with patients with muscular tension having greater forearm EMG activity (4–14 Hz) and frontalis EMG activity (14–90 Hz) than other patients, and those with mainly headache symptoms having greater muscle tension than controls (Fig. 4.7), but there were also contradictory findings (headache group having greater skin conductance, cardiac group having the lowest heart rate). This shows that the measurement of an anxious symptom is not a firm predictor of the underlying physiological state.

Despite these findings it would be wrong to disregard the physical symptoms of an anxious patient as mere outpourings of a troubled soul that have no physiological basis. In Fig. 4.8, the results of a comparison

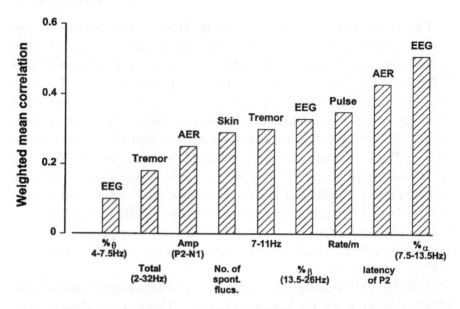

Fig. 4.8 Correlations between physiological measures and anxious mood in 32 normal subjects tested on 10 occasions during induced anxiety and rest. NB. The correlations have all been shown as positive ones for convenience. However, the associations for EEG activity (θ and α, but not β) are negative ones, as is the latency of peak 2 (P2) of the auditory evoked response, as this is generally reduced in anxiety.

between the anxious mood of 32 normal subjects tested on 10 occasions, both at rest and during induced anxiety from a variety of stimuli and underlying physiological changes, are shown. Within subject, correlations between a self-rated anxiety factor (derived from a 16 item mood scale) (Bond and Lader, 1974) and the relevant physiological measure were combined using Fisher's z-transformation. Significant and meaningful correlations were shown between the anxiety factor and many measures, with central measurements generally showing higher correlations than peripheral ones (Tyrer and Lader, 1976). It is worth noting that heart rate, a simple measure to record, is reasonably well correlated with anxiety and may often be preferred to more sophisticated measures. Physiological activity within the alpha frequency range is also highly correlated with anxiety for both the EEG and tremor.

CENTRAL GENERATION OF ANXIETY

Why do we become anxious in some situation but remain calm in others and why is there so much variation between individuals in feeling anxiety? In order to answer these questions we need first to be aware that anxiety is a symptom of great biological significance; normal anxiety is no more than ordinary prudence which helps to preserve life and protect the species. In this respect, it is not surprising that anxiety is generally much more common in women than in men in most societies of the world; women generally have to carry not only the preservation of themselves but also of their children to a much greater extent then men.

Several processes take place before a stimulus or situation creates anxiety. In man, a large number of these take place through the intervention of the cortex, but it is interesting that anxiety is remarkably similar in expression throughout the animal kingdom and it is only in man and the mammals in which the cortex plays a major part in this expression.

PERCEPTION OF THREAT

In order for someone to become anxious, there usually needs to be threat perceived in the immediate environment. There are some exceptions, of which the best known is the symptom of panic in which sudden attacks of anxiety occur without any apparent stimulus and are entirely unpredictable.

After perception of threat, the next stage is the identification of its source. Like all physiological systems, there is a desire to preserve the status quo and correct any imbalance. Action of some sort will usually be necessary to counteract the threat and return the person to a state of harmony again. Of course, in many cases it is not possible to identify the source of the threat clearly. This is most commonly expressed in the term "free-floating anxiety" to describe the anxiety of generalised anxiety disorder in which there is a general feeling of unease and danger in all situations. In other instances, the anxiety is clearly focused on a specific stimulus, and in this context, is often described as fear.

PHYSIOLOGICAL MECHANISMS INVOLVED IN PERCEPTION OF THREAT

The perception of threat is critical to the expression of anxiety. It is also important for all organisms to have systems which identify threat successfully so that they can take appropriate action. In understanding the changes that take place in the brain ensuring the perception of threat, it is valuable to know that anxiety is a primitive emotion that is expressed in similar ways throughout the animal kingdom. Much of our current knowledge is derived from studies in other mammals, notably the rat, which although lacking all the information derived form higher orders of consciousness, is nonetheless an extremely good paradigm for understanding anxiety in man.

An important and influential theory to explain how threat and anxiety are linked has been provided by Jeffery Gray (1976, 1982). Gray's work has largely been carried out in the rat which has a well defined septo-hippocampal system, which is an important part of the limbic system that has long been realised to be the "seat of the emotions" (McLean, 1955). The septum is much more highly developed in the rat than in man but the principles of Gray's theory apply equally to man.

Gray's model is a cybernetic model that is difficult to prove or disprove, although it seems likely that with the introduction of positive emission tomography (PET) in scans and other imaging techniques to record brain changes during emotional states, proof of this theory might be forthcoming. In simple terms, Gray perceives the septo-hippocampal system as a computer that is constantly monitoring the input of information from external and internal stimuli. As the afferent pathway to the brain passes through or very close to the septo-hippocampal system, it is admirably placed to carry out such a monitoring process (Fig. 4.9).

For most of the time, the system operates in "checking" mode in which the actual incoming stimuli are compared with the expected stimuli. Under normal circumstances, there will be a good match between what stimuli are expected and what actually arrive and, under these circumstances, the septo-hippocampal system still operates in checking mode. Under these circumstances, the efferent pathways concerned

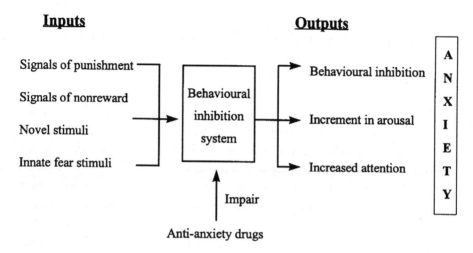

Fig. 4.9 The behavioural inhibition system according to Gray (1982). The system responds to any of its adequate inputs with all of its outputs.

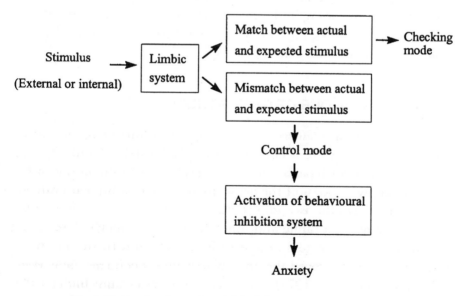

Fig. 4.10 Gray's cybernetic model of the generation of anxiety.

with the expression of anxiety and other emotions are not activated and remain quiet.

If there is a discrepancy between the expected and actual stimuli, the septo-hippocampal system becomes disturbed. If the mismatch continues for any significant length of time (and this may be only a few seconds in emergency situations), the system operates in "control" mode. In this mode, the sympathetic nervous system and efferent pathways to the "emotional" part of the cortex are activated and, in simple language, the alarm is raised. This is the time in which anxiety becomes expressed as both an emotion and a physical symptom.

Gray has termed this circuit the "behavioural inhibition system", which although at first appearing to contradict the general notion that anxiety is associated with an increase in activity, is aptly described in the rat. A non-anxious rat will explore its surroundings, groom itself, and indulge in a range of exploratory activity. When it becomes anxious, however, it "freezes" and so it is easy to see that anxiety has inhibited the normal pattern of behaviour.

The septo-hippocampal system continues operating in control mode for as long as incoming and expected stimuli remain discordant, but when they return to equilibrium the system also returns to check mode again and anxiety immediately lessens.

EVIDENCE IN FAVOUR OF GRAY'S THEORY

Until recently the main experiments supporting physiological theories and mechanisms were a combination of stimulation and ablation experiments, in which parts of transfitting systems were either stimulated or inhibited by removal of the active pathway. There is good evidence that stimulation of the ascending pathways from the septo-hippocampal gyrus to the median raphe and other structural pathways close to the fourth ventricle leads to an increase in anxiety, and conversely, when these tracts are destroyed the anxiety becomes much less (Gray *et al.*, 1976, 1982, Tye *et al.*, 1977). However, this does not test the essential cybernetic elements of the proposed theory; the matching of expected and actual stimuli which is central to the theory.

There is also a great deal of neuropharmacological evidence that is worth discussing here. Some of it can be used to support Gray's theory; some of it follows different lines. What is clear is that there are many pharmacological models of anxiety that might be useful in understanding anxiety in general (Charney and Redmond, 1983), and the anxiety of post-panic in particular (Charney *et al.*, 1985; Charney *et al.*, 1987; Charney and Deutch, 1996). Drugs such as yohimbine and caffeine can induce changes so similar to panic they are indistinguishable; further work linking this to the neurophysiology of normal anxiety may be one of the most productive avenues of research in the next decade.

Chapter 5

CLASSIFICATION OF ANXIETY

"In many cases the so-called 'anxiety conditions' gradually come on; one scarcely ever sees a case of advanced neurasthenia without the existence of some form of 'anxiety'. In the simpler forms of anxiety (nosophobia), there may be only a fear of impending insanity or of approaching death or of apoplexy. More frequently the anxious feeling is located somewhere in the body — in the praecordial region, in the head, in the abdomen, in the thorax, or more rarely in the extremities. In some cases the anxiety becomes intense and the patients are restless, and declare that they do not know what to do with themselves. They may throw themselves upon a bed, crying and complaining, and making various convulsive movement with the hands and feet. Suicidal tendencies are not uncommon in such cases, and the patient may in desperation actually take their own lives. Involuntary mental activity may be troublesome. Sometimes a patient complains that a definite word, a name, a number, a melody, or a song keeps running in his head in spite of all he can do to abolish it. In the severer cases the so-called 'phobias' are common. The most frequent form perhaps is agoraphobia, in which patients the moment they come into an open space are oppressed by an exaggerated feeling of anxiety. The fear of people and society is known as anthropophobia. A whole series of other phobias have been described — batophobia, or feelings that high things will fall; pathophobia, or fear of disease, siderodromophobia, or fear of a railway journey; siderophobia and astrophobia, fear of thunder and lightning. Occasionally we meet with individuals who are afraid of everything and everyone — victims of the so-called pantophobia."

William Osler, 1912

This account of anxiety, which at the time was all classified under the general heading of neurasthenia, a condition in which there was a deficiency of "nerve force", includes all the disorders — panic, generalised anxiety, somatoform disorders, obsessive compulsive disorder and phobias — which together now make up the anxiety disorders in the current psychiatric classification. It is always useful to be reminded that there is nothing new under the sun and Osler's account demonstrates this very well.

In the name of progress, we often split up groups that were formerly aggregated and this is true of anxiety in the current classification. Symptoms of anxiety are coded according to their quality and severity, defined using a carefully honed operational criteria, and pigeon-holed accordingly. A good classification is one that is useful (Kendell, 1989) and usefulness depends on who the user is. Classifications in psychiatry are mainly for clinicians and their view carries the greatest weight. However, there are others who also have a legitimate interest in the classification of anxiety and their views may not always agree with those of the clinicians'. Ideally, however, all users would agree with an ideal classification that "carves nature at its joints" and thereby creates a set of conditions that all who use the classification, whatever their orientation, agree is the best available. In discussing and dissecting the classification of anxiety, it is important to realise that classification in all parts of psychiatry remains a rudimentary discipline. Psychiatrists have long looked in vain for a new Linnaeus to come and identify the central element which could serve as the common backbone to the classification system. Linnaeus founded it in sex, but despite psychiatrists' preoccupation with this subject, it has been a hopeless classifier. After flirting with the psychodynamic concepts of unconscious motivations, defence and denial, and physical explanations such as focal sepsis and different forms of brain disease, psychiatry has settled back to the somewhat uneasy compromise of classifying disorders by attempting to define the symptoms and behaviour associated with them clearly and unequivocally. Such a classification system is atheoretical; it has no prior conceptions and might best be summed up in the computer programmer's acronym, WYSIWYG (What You See Is What You Get).

Although this exercise can be useful, it is really more of a pre-classification system than a real one. A geographer from Mars could carry out a perfectly good WYSIWYG classification of the earth through serial observations to compensate for cloud cover. He would be able to identify the cold and warm regions of the planet, the land and the sea, the mountains and the valleys, the jungles and the deserts, and climatic variations with the season. This would be extremely valuable from the strictly topographical viewpoint but would tell us nothing at all about life on earth. You would have to make interpretations from these data to reach the conclusion that life existed on earth, and would have to go even further, mainly by identifying the Great Wall of China, the firebreaks that extend for hundreds of miles between the forests of northern Canada, and large open caste mines in countries such as Australia, to conclude that there was intelligent life on earth. The WYSIWYG approach gives the bare outlines only; it has the benefit of accuracy, but without interpretation and refinement, its value is limited.

The classification of anxiety illustrates all the advantages and disadvantages of the WYSIWYG approach. Anxiety can present in various forms; these can be identified and to some extent delineated, and the resulting classification has face validity. It is when we attempt to interpret and extrapolate from this classification that the difficulties emerge.

The existing classification of anxiety disorders is summarised in Table 5.1. This includes the diagnostic codes of the two major classification systems of psychiatry, the International Classification of Diseases (ICD), now in its tenth revision (World Health Organisation, 1992) and the Diagnostic and Statistical Manual for Mental Disorders (DSM) the United States classification that has achieved widespread popularity in many countries of the world, and is now in its fourth revision (American Psychiatric Association, 1994).

It is worth following the classification from the point of view of the patient as we ask each of them questions in the flowchart shown in Table 5.1. The first question separates those with what could be described as "constitutional anxiety" from those who have "stress anxiety". Although there is often considerable overlap between them, the importance of making this distinction in treatment is so strong that the stress and adjustment disorders have to be identified as early as possible.

Table 5.1 Classification of Anxiety Disorders

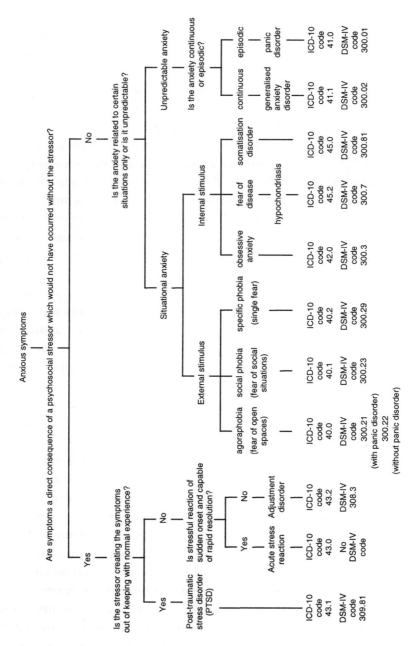

STRESS AND ADJUSTMENT DISORDERS

These conditions, particularly post-traumatic stress disorder, have become increasingly prominent in recent years, and have been fuelled by media and medicolegal interest, particularly in respect of post-traumatic stress disorder. When a diagnosis achieves the spotlight in an area which it was never meant to illuminate, it is reasonable to question whether its original purpose has been perverted.

There are three forms of stress disorder in which anxiety is a prominent symptom: acute stress reactions, adjustment disorders and post-traumatic stress disorder. Acute stress reactions are identified in ICD-10 as symptoms typical of generalised anxiety disorder (autonomic symptoms such as sweating and palpitations, respiratory and abdominal symptoms, dizziness and fears of losing control, tension and irritability), together with other symptoms or behaviour indicating distress, such as disorientation, reduced attention, anger, despair, inappropriate overactivity and excessive grief. It is only classified in ICD-10 and some might dispute its value, as, by definition, "the symptoms must begin to diminish after no more than 8 hours" if the stress is removed, or no more than 48 hours if the stress continues. The stressor has to be "an exceptional mental or physical" one and symptoms should begin with one hour of exposure. In short, the main symptoms are basically those of normal anxiety.

Adjustment disorders are slower to develop (occurrence within one month of exposure to stressor) and longer-lasting (up to two years) but no longer than six months after the stress has disappeared, and can include symptoms of any mood, neurotic or conduct disorders. They are further subdivided into brief (< one month) and prolonged depressive disorders (up to two years) (in ICD-10 only); anxiety (including separation anxiety); other emotions; disturbances of conduct (e.g. violence, truancy, vandalism); and mixed emotions and conduct. As the advertisement for one of our well-known tabloid newspapers has it, all human life is there in the world of adjustment disorders.

One of the major deficiencies in our knowledge of anxiety is the significance of the symptom in the context of adjustment disorder. There are likely to be important differences in the nature of this type of anxiety and all the other conditions discussed in this book. It may be that these differences are only those between normal and pathological anxiety discussed in Chapters 1 and 10, but it is likely that there is more to adjustment anxiety than this. One possible clue is the high rate of personality disorders found in patients with adjustment disorder. This is extremely high, with a rate of 50% in one study (Tyrer *et al.*, 1988), significantly higher than the rate with anxiety states (39.6%) and with a preponderance of dependent and impulsive personality characteristics. Other work suggests that people with these personality disorders create, rather than merely respond to, adverse life events (Seivewright, 1987; Seivewright *et al.*, 1998, to be published); and this may account for the high prevalence of personality disorders in patients with adjustment disorders.

Post-traumatic stress disorder is currently one of the most fashionable diagnoses in psychiatry and one in which anxiety is usually the most prominent symptom. The main criteria for the diagnosis in ICD-10 and DSM-IV are shown in Table 5.2. It does not take much thought to realise that the only important criterion for the diagnosis is the first one — exposure to an exceptional stressor — the others are mixtures of generalised anxiety, panic symptoms, phobic avoidance and dissociation (the condition formerly described as hysteria in which unpleasant symptoms are denied in part or completely so there is selective memory loss).

This may seem like carping criticism but needs to be stated because so many have fallen in love with post-traumatic stress disorder as a new and exciting diagnosis that represents an important breakthrough (Ramsay, 1990). It was first formulated as a psychiatric diagnosis by Kardiner in 1941 and its main features can be identified from old accounts, one of the most celebrated being Samuel Pepys' description of the effects of the Great Fire of London (Daly, 1983). Anxiety is a great mimic, and the identification of a disorder in such clear fashion from operational criteria is highly relevant in post-traumatic stress disorder because of its medico-legal significance. Put yourself in the shoes of a person who has experienced a major disaster such as a large fire in a crowded building leading to serious injury of at least one person. If this

Table 5.2 Diagnostic Criteria for Post-traumatic Stress Disorder

Feature	ICD-10	DSM-IV
Nature	Exposure to an extremely threatening stressful event	
Symptoms	Repeated re-living of the trauma in intrusive flashbacks, vivid memories, or recurring dreams. Stress is experienced when there is exposure to circumstances reminiscent of the trauma There is fear and avoidance of circumstances resembling or associated with the trauma Either of the following must be present 1. Inability to recall, either partially or completely, some important aspects of the period of exposure to the stressor 2. Persistent symptoms of increased psychological sensitivity and arousal (not present before exposure to stressor), and by any two of the following (a) difficulty in falling or staying asleep (b) irritability and outbursts of anger (c) difficulty in concentrating (d) hypervigilance (e) exaggerated startle response	Traumatic event is persistently re-experienced in at least one of the following ways 1. Recurrent and intrusive recollections of the event 2. Recurrent distressing dreams of the event 3. Sudden feeling as if the traumatic event were recurring (including sense of reliving the experiences, illusions, hallucinations and dissociative [flashback] episodes) 4. Intense psychological distress at exposure to events that symbolise the traumatic event e.g. anniversaries of the trauma Persistent avoidance of stimuli associated with the trauma and numbing of general responsiveness (not present before the trauma). Three or more of the following must be shown 1. Efforts to avoid thoughts, or feelings associated with the trauma 2. Efforts to avoid activities, or situations that arouse recollections of the trauma 3. Inability to recall an important aspect of the trauma 4. Markedly diminished interest in significant activities 5. Feelings of detachment or estrangement from others 6. Restricted range of affect (e.g. unable to have loving feelings) 7. Sense of foreshortened future Persistent symptoms of increased arousal (not present before the trauma), shown by at least two of the following 1. difficulty in falling or staying asleep 2. irritability and outbursts of anger 3. difficulty in concentrating 4. hypervigilance 5. exaggerated startle response 6. physiologic reactivity upon exposure to events that symbolise the traumatic event
Onset and duration	Should only be diagnosed if condition has arisen within six months of the stressful event. Very occasionally onset may be delayed.	At least one month Delayed onset if onset of symptoms was at least six months after the trauma

person has had experience of pathological anxiety in the past (and very few of us have not at some stage), the exhibition of all the symptoms of post-traumatic stress disorder could be developed in a few days and, if someone can be held responsible, legal action will start shortly afterwards. All that is needed is a pleasant psychiatrist or psychologist to accord the diagnosis of post-traumatic stress disorder and the case is cut and dried.

This can develop in many people without any inkling of bad faith, lying or malingering. Anxiety has epidemic qualities and the symptoms can be generated even by reading press accounts of the incident — "I didn't realise it was as bad as that; I think I'm going to have a panic" — or talking to others who have developed symptoms after the event. Any continuing media interest can further fuel any existing anxiety and reinforce the pattern. Woe betide any expert who questions the veracity of this account or suggests it might have turned out differently if others had not magnified the implications of the event. "Someone 'as got to be summonsed, and that was decided upon", as Stanley Holloway declaimed in his Lancashire ditty on *Albert and the Lion,* and any number of other experts can be rounded up to parrot the diagnostic criteria of post-traumatic stress disorder and show that the poor sufferer unquestionably has all the symptoms *and would never have had them but for the exceptionally stressful event* (I put the last part in italics to show the arrogance of some experts who seem able to summarise an individual's life moods on the basis of a single interview).

Post-traumatic stress disorder undoubtedly exists, and some of its best descriptions come from the articles of Frederick Mott of casualties from the First World War (Mott, 1918). What is of great concern is that the main features, or more accurately, a hotchpotch of symptoms (which are now so well-known they can be downloaded from the Internet), now substitute for a careful assessment of all the features, both genuine pathology and induced extras, and make a charade of diagnosis.

SITUATIONAL ANXIETY

Following the procedure outlined in Table 5.1, the next group of disorders to be considered in the classification is those anxiety disorders which are not stress or adjustment disorders but which are responses to identifiable stimuli. In these instances the response may be excessive but the stimulus is clear. Anxiety which is clearly linked to an external stimulus is situational anxiety, which is almost, but not quite, encapsulated in the word "fear", and which introduces us to the subject of phobias.

Phobias were first identified as psychiatric disorders in 1871 by Westphal, who introduced the term "agoraphobia" or fear of the market place, to characterise the anxiety of people who were generally calm in

Table 5.3 Diagnostic Criteria for the Three Main Groups of Phobias

Type of phobia	ICD-10	DSM-IV
Agoraphobia (with or without history of panic disorder)	Fear of leaving home, remaining at home alone, entering shops, crowds and public places, or travelling alone in trains, buses or planes	Fear of being in places from which escape is difficult or embarrassing. Situations are avoided or endured with marked distress. If panic attacks present diagnosis is Agoraphobia with Panic Disorder, alternatively it is Agoraphobia without Panic Disorder
Social phobia	Fear of scrutiny by other people in comparatively small groups (i.e. not crowds). (Symptoms may progress to panic attacks)	Fear of being in social situation because of close scrutiny by others and fear of possible humiliation or embarrassment
Specific phobia (specific or isolated phobias in ICD)	Fear of "highly specific object or situation" including animals, birds, insects, heights, thunder, flying, small enclosed spaces, the sight of blood or injury, injections, dentists and hospitals. Symptoms of anxiety (as for GAD and Panic) must have been present at some time in the feared situation and/or have led to avoidance. Distress caused by symptoms or avoidance.	Marked and persistent fear that is excessive and unreasonable, cued by presence or anticipation of a "specific object or situation" (examples as for ICD-10), which almost invariably produces an anxiety response (including panic sometimes) and which interferes with normal routine.

their own homes but anxious when out of doors, particularly in busy streets, markets, open spaces and public transport. Any situation in which the person felt powerless was likely to be incorporated into the phobia. The term caught on quickly and before long graeco-latin epithets for all types of phobia were introduced; some of these are illustrated in the quotation from William Osler at the beginning of this chapter (p. 80). Before long, this approach to description was seen to be little more than linguistic showing off; nothing was gained apart from a new word to the language by describing phobias in this way.

Most of the phobias so identified were well encapsulated in nature and could all be incorporated under the heading of simple or specific phobias. The other two types of phobia worthy of separate identification were social phobia and agoraphobia. The current criteria for their classification are shown in Table 5.3. The key elements in differentiating them are the fear of being out of doors in a variety of strange uncontrolled situations (agoraphobia), the fear of being observed and scrutinised by others (social phobia) and the fear of well demarcated objects, animals or situations that can generally be predicted and avoided (simple phobia).

AGORAPHOBIA

Agoraphobia, like all phobias, involves both the fear of being in places or situations and avoidance of such situations as a result of the fear. These situations are diffuse and normally experienced by people at least daily; avoidance and fear of such situations therefore leads to substantial handicap. Agoraphobia is normally more severe in its impact on life than other phobias and is often associated with complications such as depression and melancholia (Breier *et al.*, 1984; Lesser *et al.*, 1988), particularly when it is severe (Chambless, 1985). Although it is hallowed by long use, the concept still has its critics, as people with severe anxiety of whatever type are not likely to expose themselves to situations which only increase their anxiety. The notion that the typical agoraphobic stays at home in calm and tranquillity and is suddenly changed to nervous jelly on stepping out of the front door is far from the truth (Hallam, 1978).

Where matters become complicated with agoraphobia is when we consider the position of panic. Panic disorder as a diagnosis in its own right is described later, but, unlike almost every other diagnosis in DSM-IV, it is accorded co-diagnostic status with agoraphobia. This privilege is not accorded to social phobia or post-traumatic stress disorder, conditions in which panic is at least as prevalent as agoraphobia. It is largely because of the work of Donald Klein, who argued that panic was a common precursor of agoraphobia and had a major influence on its development and perpetuation, that agoraphobia with panic has become a single diagnostic entity. Of course, this leaves us with the diagnosis of agoraphobia without panic disorder (often abbreviated to AWOPD), which is common in non-clinical populations (Weissman, 1985) and which differs in several ways from agoraphobia with panic. For example, patients with agoraphobia without panic are more likely to have generalised anxiety disorder and avoidant personality disorder, and those with agoraphobia with panic to have obsessive-compulsive disorder and alcohol dependence (Hoffart *et al.*, 1995), suggesting that the panic group are less well and more socially distressed.

SOCIAL PHOBIA

Social phobia is characterised by the fear of being scrutinised by others and humiliated because of apparent inadequacies in appearance, speech or performance in various ways (Marks, 1970). As befits the Yerkes-Dodson curve, such anxiety tends to impair performance and so, even if the ideas of inadequacy are unjustified, they become true in practice because anxiety, the grand saboteur, evokes its own humiliation. It has become recognised as an increasingly important disorder in recent years, mainly following evidence of its high prevalence in the United States in particular (2.6% lifetime prevalence) (Kessler *et al.*, 1994), the degree of social impairment created by the condition (Schneier *et al.*, 1994) and the fact that the condition appears to precede other psychiatric disorders (usually in adolescence), which has implications for prevention (Kessler *et al.*, 1996).

Despite its frequency, only one in 20 of those with "pure" social phobia had sought treatment for the condition, and this needs some explanation. One could be that the act of consultation with the condition is itself socially phobic, so patients regard the doctor's surgery as a phobic situation. Another could be the perception that nothing can be done to help it, and a third could be a diagnostic one, that the condition is confused with avoidant personality disorder in particular, and therefore, may be misdiagnosed. Whatever the explanation, the subject is likely to assume a greater profile than formerly.

SPECIFIC PHOBIA

These conditions are also very common (prevalence of around 8%) (Agras et al., 1969) and many belong with normal anxiety despite being accorded the code of a psychiatric diagnosis. Many are not associated with any major social disruption as avoiding action can be taken without much difficulty. Thus a phobia of mice is not normally a problem as in the average working week a mouse will rarely be encountered. It is only when the expectations of living involve exposure to the phobia on a regular basis that problems sufficient for clinical intervention are created.

The treatment of specific or simple phobias is one of the major successes of psychological treatment in psychiatry. Systematic desensitisation and exposure therapy are remarkably effective in not only alleviating, but often eliminating, both fears and avoidance, in people with fears of needles (Ferguson et al., 1978), heights (Baker et al., 1973) and a range of other conditions (Watson et al., 1972). By contrast, pharmacological treatments such as imipramine are ineffective (Zitrin et al., 1983). There is less discussion of this subject in this book than might be justified because most of the people with these disorders are really from "non-clinical populations", a somewhat unfortunate phrase which many appear to minimise handicap, but one which really indicates that very few of these come into contact with ordinary practice either in primary or secondary care.

SOMATOFORM DISORDERS

These disorders cover a range of conditions in which a psychiatric disorder is considered to be present but in which the major symptoms are those of physical disorder. It could be argued that these are not part of the anxiety spectrum but separate neurotic disorders. In the past they were regarded as part of the spectrum of hysteria, whereby unacceptable anxiety was converted into acceptable physical disorder. Now that it has been recognised that the anxiety orchestra has many instruments, some of which are entirely from the bodily section, it has become accepted that many of the symptoms of physical disease exhibited by psychiatric patients are genuine and have a proper physiological basis (see Chapter 4). This does not mean that they are all explicable in physiological terms and the variation between the different diagnoses in this group is accounted for to a much greater extent by mental state and cognitive variables than by physiological ones.

The tendency to express symptoms in physical form is known as somatisation and the range of morbid anxiety encompasses the extremes of both 100% somatisation and 100% expression of psychological symptoms (Fig. 5.1). Only the somatoform disorders concentrate all their

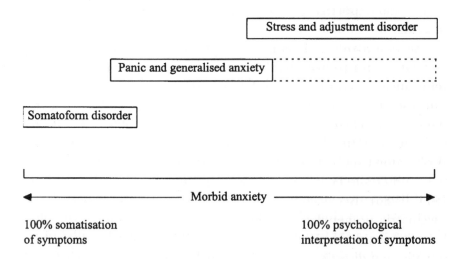

Fig. 5.1 The spectrum of somatoform and anxiety disorders.

features at the somatic section of the spectrum; other psychiatric disorders have marked somatic and bodily symptoms but do not focus their attention on these exclusively. At the other extreme, we have the conditions in which most of the distress is psychological; most of the typical anxiety disorders include both somatic and pychological aspects but in milder form can extend towards 100% "psychologising". A good definition of somatisation is that by Lipowski (1988): "a tendency to experience and communicate somatic distress and other symptoms unaccounted for by pathological findings, to attribute them to physical illness and to seek medical help for them".

There are many reasons why patients may somatise but none of them has yet proved to be of special value. What is clear is that anxiety is closely associated with somatisation and is found more commonly in persistent somatisers than any other psychiatric disorder (Fink, 1995). Because somatisers are extremely reluctant to admit any degree of psychological causation for their symptoms, such anxiety is almost invariably attributed to worry over the apparent physical disorder rather than a primary phenomenon. This explains why the justification for their symptoms is always perceived as an internal rather than any external one (Table 5.1).

The two important groups of somatoform disorder are somatisation disorder, the ultimate somatising phenomenon, in which attention is focused on a wide range of organ systems in the body, and this is associated with persistence of symptoms, often over many years, and reluctance to accept that there is no medical cause for the condition. This used to be known as Briquet's syndrome, named after the French physician who first reported this condition 150 years ago, but which was defined and refined by the work of Samuel Guze and his colleagues in Washington University School of Medicine, St Louis, Missouri, who found the condition to be incredibly stable over a long time scale (Guze *et al.*, 1971; 1986). Because this new condition replaced hysteria in the psychiatric nomenclature (Guze, 1967), it is often called "St Louis hysteria" as a nod to its predecessor. The main problem associated with somatisation disorder for health services is the excessive use of medical services for unnecessary investigations. The persistent use of such services

Table 5.4 Diagnostic Characteristics of Somatoform Disorders

ICD-10	DSM-IV
Somatization disorder: multiple and variable physical symptoms that cannot be explained by any detectable physical disorders, associated with preoccupation and distress and which leads to patient to seek repeated (three or more) consultations or sets of investigations with doctors (either in primary or secondary care). Persistent refusal to accept medical reassurance that there is no adequate physical cause for symptoms. Six or more of following symptoms:- abdominal pain, nausea, bloated feelings, bad taste, vomiting, loose bowels, chest pains, breathlessness, dysuria, genital discomfort, vaginal discharge, blotchy skin, limb or joint pain, numbness	Somatization disorder: history of many physical complaints beginning before the age of 30 occurring over several years, for which medical attention has been sought, but which are not due to any physical disorder. The symptoms must include at least 4 pain symptoms (pain relating to at least 4 different sites or functions), two gastrointestinal symptoms (nausea, vomiting, bloating, diarrhoea, food intolerance), one sexual symptom (e.g. sexual indifference, erectile dysfunction) and one pseudoneurological symptom e.g. difficulty in swallowing, aphonia)
Hypochondriacal syndrome: persistent preoccupation with a possibility of having a maximum of two physical diseases, manifest by persistent distress and interference in daily living; persistent refusal to accept medical reassurance that there is no physical cause for symptoms	Somatoform pain disorder: preoccupation with pain in the absence of adequate physical findings to account for it
	Hypochondriasis: preoccupation with the fear of having, or the belief that one has, a serious disease without evidence of this on physical evaluation
Body dysmorphic disorder, as described in DSM-IV but included as a form of hypochondriacal disorder	Body Dysmorphic Disorder (dysmorphophobia): preoccupation with imagined defect in appearance, causing significant distress, and not better accounted for by another mental disorder
Dissociative (conversion) disorders: Characteristic (motor or sensory) disorder that cannot be explained by physical disorder; can be shown as amnesia, fugue, stupor, trance and possession disorders, motor disorders, convulsions, anaesthesia or sensory loss, and mixed disorders	Conversion disorder: one or more symptoms or deficits affecting voluntary or sensory function that suggest a neurological or other general medical condition, in which psychological factors "are judged to be associated with the symptom or deficit"

and the extent to which people with this disorder will seek out such services, shows some similarities with Münchausen sydrome, the disorder first described by Richard Asher (1951) in which simulation of disease associated with persistent lying is associated with personality disorder of the flamboyant group. Somatisation disorder is also associated with this group of personalities (Guze *et al.*, 1971).

The hypochondriacal syndrome is different (Table 5.4). Although it too is persistent, and suggestions made that it may constitute a personality disorder in its own right as it represents a persistent style of behaviour (Tyrer *et al.*, 1990a), it is associated with more introverted anxious personality styles and the help-seeking behaviour is much less dramatic than in somatisation disorder. For many years, it was either assumed to be a manifestation of depression (Kenyon, 1965), and there is no doubt that hypochondriasis is a prominent component of depression (Lewis, 1934). Hypochondriasis was alternatively subsumed under "illness phobia", but is now accepted as a "stand alone" disorder (Barsky and Klerman, 1983). Only around one in five have somatisation disorder too (Barsky *et al.*, 1992) and the fundamental core of the syndrome, the suspicion that one has an undiagnosed disease, is always at the forefront of the disorder.

Two other conditions are also listed in Table 5.4 which have a more peripheral association with anxiety; body dysmorphic disorder; and conversion or dissociative disorder. Body dysmorphic disorder (formerly dysmorphophobia) describes a condition in which the sufferer becomes excessively preoccupied with a minor physical defect which either does not exist or is so minor as to be almost undetectable. This may be preoccupation over the shape of the nose, skin texture or smoothness, or the shape of the stomach. Although such preoccupations over body shape are common in anorexia nervosa, the difference in body dysmorphic disorder is that only a small part of the body is usually involved. Conversion disorder is good old-fashioned, and unequivocal, hysteria. It is the classical Freudian disorder in which anxiety over a stressful event disappears because it is "converted" into a physical disorder. Indeed, the absence of anxiety is one of the striking features of the condition, la belle indifférence, the incongruous lack of anxiety in the handicap and apparent implications of the disorder.

Obsessive anxiety is similar in some respects to hypochondriasis except that it is not always concerned with disease. Although obsessive-compulsive disorder can be separated much more successfully from other psychiatric disorders than most others in the neurotic group, there is a persistent group of obsessional thinkers (ruminators) who generate anxiety readily from their preoccupations (Goodman *et al.*, 1989) and who may account for much of the association between obsessional and anxiety disorders (Mellman and Uhde, 1987). The somewhat corny complaint from the patient "Doctor, I'm all worked up because I've got nothing to worry about" is typical of obsessive anxiety. If there is nothing to occupy the mind, it will get up to mischief and generate worrying thoughts that only generate more anxiety.

PANIC DISORDER

The flow chart of Table 5.1 shows that when no reason can be given for the onset of symptoms of anxiety (i.e. there are no obvious cues), the patient is probably suffering from panic disorder or generalised anxiety disorder. These conditions constitute the main part of morbid anxiety and are deeply distressing to patients because the source of anxiety cannot be identified (see Chapter 1).

Although panic disorder is a recently introduced member of the classification, it is worth discussing in detail because it is fundamental to the classification of anxiety. The central component of panic disorder is a panic attack and, although there is much argument over the number of panic attacks and their frequency before the diagnosis of panic disorder can be considered — the evidence suggests that frequency has little to do with the severity of disorder (Katon *et al.*, 1995) — there is little dispute over the panic attack itself. The notion of the panic attack is an ancient one; the word "panic" derives from experience suffered by travellers through the woods in ancient Greece who experienced acute attacks of anxiety when the mischievous god, Pan, jumped out in front of them or teased them in other frightening ways. The description of the panic attack as a central symptom of anxiety is also not new, and is well summarised in one of Sigmond Freud's earlier papers (Freud, 1895).

The elevation of panic from an important symptom of anxiety to a separate diagnostic group owes much to the research of one man, Donald Klein, a resourceful and inventive research worker who had a major influence on many aspects of clinical psychiatry. Klein, like many psychiatrists reared in the United States during the 1950s, was trained primarily in psychotherapy and treated most anxiety disorders by such means with the occasional use of barbiturates and hypnotics. When imipramine was introduced as a treatment for depression in the early 1960s, Klein, not unreasonably, thought it might be helpful to test the effectiveness of imipramine in anxious patients.

Anxious patients are not commonly admitted to hospital unless their symptoms are very severe and people with panic symptoms constitute a large proportion of those who do become inpatients. Klein found that imipramine was effective in these patients but not so useful in those who had more diffuse generalised anxiety. He called the first group "endogenous anxiety" and, as these patients mainly had symptoms of panic, the notion that panic disorder is equivalent to endogenous anxiety has persisted to the present day.

At this time the classification of anxiety was relatively simple but vaguely defined. Conditions in which anxiety was focused on specific situations constituted the "phobias", and when anxiety was unfocused or "free-floating" they were joined together under the general heading of "anxiety neurosis".

Klein's findings, although relatively modest in terms of numbers of patients treated, stimulated an accompanying and important notion, that of "*pharmacological dissection*". This idea is a basic one but clearly exciting if it proves to be true. Put simply, if any psychiatric disorder treated by a drug shows a clear distinction between responders and non responders, differences in the population need to be examined closely because what originally appeared to be a single disorder has been "dissected" by the drug treatment into at least two disorders. This notion is of great value to the clinician because, to go back to our earlier statement that clinical diagnosis has to be useful, any classification that allows specific treatments to be attached to it will be of great clinical value.

Thus by the end of the 1960s, the essential arguments for the establishment of panic disorder as a separate diagnosis had already been made. Panic disorder appeared to respond to antidepressants such as imipramine, whereas those with the other type of anxiety, now termed "generalised anxiety disorder" did not respond and might be better treated with sedative agents such as the benzodiazepines. Pharmacological dissection had split anxiety in the same way that psychological dissection had also been at least partly responsible for the splitting of anxiety from phobic states, as the psychological treatment of behaviour therapy could only be applied successfully when the anxiety was situational rather than diffuse.

It took several more years for panic disorder to be formally incorporated into psychiatric classification, as this was only achieved in the third revision of the *Diagnostic and Statistical Manual for Mental Disorders* in 1980 (American Psychiatric Association, 1980).

Although it might seem fairly simple to accommodate the relatively straightforward symptom of the panic attack into a psychiatric classification of panic disorder, the exercise has been fraught with difficulties. One of the initial ones encountered by Klein was that most of the patients seen with panic in psychiatric clinical practice are suffering from phobias also, particularly agoraphobia. The patient with agoraphobia has recurrent panic attacks that can prove a devastating handicap for the success of treatment such as exposure therapy (Mathews *et al.*, 1981) and when very severe, admission to hospital may be recommended. However, most panic attacks are experienced by people who have no clear cut phobic symptoms, at least initially, but neither Donald Klein nor the many other psychiatric researchers involved in the operational criteria for panic disorder in DSM-III, had any significant experience of panic attacks in these settings.

The diagnosis "agoraphobia with panic attacks" was allowed as a joint diagnosis in DSM-III, an extraordinary concession. This reflected Donald Klein's own views on the natural history about panic disorder. This was that panic disorder, in which panic attacks took place without warning, would commonly be followed by agoraphobia because the suffer naturally wished to stay in a place of safety where help was at hand rather than in an exposed environment in which physical collapse or humiliation could occur with all its attendant disasters. Agoraphobia with panic disorder was therefore expected to be the main form of agoraphobia seen in clinical practice. This expectation was supported but what was not expected was the large numbers of people seen in the community in epidemiological surveys that had agoraphobia without panic disorder but who seldom came to medical attention (Regier *et al.*, 1990a). The criteria for diagnosing a panic attack were easier to decide. A state of panic is one in which all the emergency alarm systems are operating simultaneously in the body. The sufferer experiences tremendous distress and dread and feels imminent dissolution or of going mad (see Osler's description at the beginning of this chapter), and has all the bodily accompaniment of sympathetic nervous discharge such as tremor, palpitations, difficulty in breathing, flushing and gastrointestinal symptoms (Table 5.5). To qualify for a panic attack, these symptoms have to be generated within a short time (an outer limit of 10 minutes) and also not be persistent, as physiological overdrive at this level is impossible to maintain for more than around 30 minutes at any one time.

All psychiatric classifications have categorical diagnoses, which means that separation has to be made between a low level of symptoms so that these can be placed within the range of normal function and higher levels of symptoms which are pathological. The dividing line between normal and pathological might be thought to be easier in the case of panic disorder than other conditions but this is not the case.

Another thorny issue is the relationship of the anxiety experienced in a phobic episode and panic disorder. As explained earlier, Klein's views about the relationship between panic and agoraphobia have led to the diagnosis of agoraphobia with panic disorder being given separate diagnostic status in DSM-III, but, despite the fact that panic disorder can also co-exist with social phobia, such a combined diagnosis was not considered when both these were present at the same time. The problem becomes more complicated when one considers the intense anxiety that can be experienced by phobic patients in their phobic situations. The key question is whether such anxiety is unpredictable. If a panic attack is experienced every time a person enters the phobic situation, it cannot be regarded as predictable, but if it only occurs on one occasion in five,

Table 5.5 Diagnostic Criteria for Panic Disorder

Feature	ICD-10	DSM-IV
Duration and setting	Recurrent unexpected panic attacks which are often spontaneous and unpredictable. They are not associated with marked exertion or with exposure to dangerous situations	
Symptoms	Discrete period of intense fear. Starts abruptly — reaches maximum within a few minutes and lasts at least some minutes. One from the first four symptoms and at least three others present Autonomic arousal symptoms 1. Palpitations, pounding heart or accelerated heart rate 2. Sweating 3. Trembling or shaking 4. Dry mouth Other symptoms Difficulty in breathing Choking feeling Chest pain or discomfort Nausea or abdominal distress Feeling dizzy, unsteady, faint or lightheaded Derealisation (feeling of unreality) Depersonalisation (being detached from oneself) Fear of losing control, going crazy Fear of dying Hot flushes or cold chills Numbness or tingling sensations	A discrete period of intense fear in which four or more of the following symptoms develop abruptly and reach a peak within 10 minutes: Palpitations, pounding heart or accelerated heart rate Sweating Trembling or shaking Sensation of shortness of breath or smothering Choking feeling Chest pain or discomfort Nausea or abdominal distress Feeling dizzy, unsteady, faint or lightheaded Derealisation (feeling of unreallity) Depersonalisation (being detached from oneself) Fear of losing control, going crazy Fear of dying Hot flushes or cold chills Numbness or tingling sensations Recurrent unexpected panic attacks. At least one of the attacks has been followed by one month or more of at least one of the following: (a) Concern about having more attacks (b) Worry about implication of the attack (c) A significant change in behaviour related to the panic attacks
Exclusion criteria	Panic attacks not due to physical disorder, organic mental disorder, or other mental disorders such as schizophrenia and other related disorders, mood [affective] disorders, or somatoform disorders.	Panic attacks not due to the direct effects of a substance (e.g. drug of abuse, medication or general medical condition). Other mental disorders such as social phobia, obsessive compulsive disorder, post-traumatic stress disorder and separation anxiety disorder must also be excluded.

is the condition better described as panic disorder or as phobic anxiety? Neither classification gives a satisfactory answer to this question and work on panic disorders in natural environments has shown that patients' personal accounts of their panics may often be unreliable (Margraf et al., 1987).

Attempts have also been made at different times to include an intermediate level of panic disorder with limited phobic avoidance (Sheehan, 1983), and moderate panic disorder (at least four panic attacks in a four week period (code F41.00 in ICD-10), although what one might feel is the mildest form of panic disorders, the single panic attack, is not given a code classification in DSM-IV despite being carefully defined. This range indicates that panic covers a continuum of symptoms; not even the apparent all-or-none phenomenon of the panic attack can avoid the indignity of being graded in severity.

There have also been suggestions that panic disorder can be separated into a group which has primary respiratory symptoms such as choking sensations, difficulty in breathing and hyperventilation, and panic disorder with other bodily symptoms (Briggs et al., 1993). The distinction could, in principle, be an important one because it is claimed that the respiratory group are more likely to respond to apresoline while the other responds better to antidepressants such as imipramine (Briggs et al., 1993). These claims require verification from other studies. Finally, there is also a distinction claimed for primary and secondary panic disorder (Starcevic et al., 1993) which requires further substantiation.

What must be clear to the reader is that panic disorder is a very powerful and influential diagnosis that is moving forward very quickly; indeed, as one recent writer has reported, "an attempt to write a book on the topic is rather like trying to describe a moving train as it roars past" (Baker, 1989). However, like all trains, it will eventually arrive at its terminus and it may not be as impressive when stationary as on the move.

GENERALISED ANXIETY DISORDER

Generalised anxiety disorder is not really a positive diagnosis; it tends to be given to patients who do not qualify for other specific diagnoses of anxiety but who still clearly have anxiety symptoms. The criteria listed in Table 5.6 suggests otherwise (particularly the overlap with panic disorder in DSM-IV); there are some distinctions between the symptoms of generalised anxiety disorder and other conditions (more in DSM-IV than ICD-10), but in clinical practice GAD (its common abbreviation) is an anxiety dustbin for rejected patients. Nosological dustbins tend to be full of heterogeneous patients and this is certainly true of generalised anxiety disorder (Hoehn-Saric, 1985; Brawman-Mintzer *et al.*, 1993).

The symptoms of generalised anxiety disorder are quantitatively less marked than those of panic disorder but in other respects are not very different (Hoehn-Saric, 1982; Anderson *et al.*, 1984; Hoehn-Saric and McLeod, 1985; Starcevic *et al.*, 1994), and rather pointedly in the ICD-10 criteria, are exactly the same. There are, however, arguments that the conditions respond to different treatments even though this does not approach pharmacological or psychological dissection (Barlow *et al.*, 1984). The essential elements of both somatic (bodily) and psychological components of anxiety, are easily identified in the three sets of criteria for the diagnosis and, as with all operational criteria, a somewhat arbitrary decision has to be made about the number of symptoms qualifying for the diagnosis in each group.

The duration of symptoms before the diagnosis of GAD can be made is set at six months during which period symptoms have to be experienced on most days. This may seem reasonable but can lead to problems when diagnoses are compared and when comorbidity is examined (see Chapter 9). Panic disorder can be diagnosed after only a few days, major depression after two weeks, generalised anxiety disorder after six months and dysthymic disorder (the chronic form of what used to be called "depressive neurosis") after two years. This temporal juggling does not gain respect for the classification of these disorders and leads to severe problems when one tries to decide which diagnosis takes precedence (Boyd *et al.*, 1984).

One of the major difficulties in defining the lower diagnostic boundary of GAD is the overlap with anxious or avoidant personality disorder. This diagnosis is discussed later in this chapter but the key clinical distinction between the two is whether the symptoms can be regarded as intrinsic to that person's normal functioning (or egosyntonic according

Table 5.6 Diagnostic Criteria for the Diagnosis of Generalised Anxiety Disorder

Feature	ICD-10	DSM-IV
Duration and setting	Excessive anxiety, worry and tension occurring more days than not for at least six months with feelings of apprehension about everyday events or activities	
Symptoms	One from the first four symptoms and at least three others must be present	The anxiety and worry are associated with three or more of the following six symptoms (with at least some of them being present more days than not for the last six months)
	Autonomic arousal symptoms 1. Palpitations, pounding heart or accelerated heart rate 2. Sweating 3. Trembling or shaking 4. Dry mouth	1. Restlessness, feeling keyed up or on edge 2. Being easily fatigued 3. Difficulty in concentrating or mind going blank 4. Irritability 5. Muscle tension 6. Sleep disturbance (difficulty falling or staying asleep, or restless unsatisfying sleep)
	Other symptoms Difficulty in breathing Choking feeling Chest pain or discomfort Nausea or abdominal distress Feeling dizzy, unsteady, faint or lightheaded Derealisation (feeling of unreality) Depersonalisation (being detached) Fear of losing control, going crazy Fear of dying Hot flushes or cold chills Numbness or tingling sensations Muscle tension or aches and pains Restlessness, unable to relax Feeling on edge, or mentally tense Sensation of a lump in the throat, or difficulty in swallowing Exaggerated response to being startled Difficulty in concentrating Persistent irritability Difficulty in sleeping	Distress or impairment in social functioning
Exclusion criteria	Anxiety disorder is not due to physical disorder (e.g. hyperthyroidism), organic mental disorder, or a psychoactive substance related disorder such as excessive amphetamine consumption or withdrawal from benzodiazepines	Anxiety disorder is not due to direct physiological effects of a substance (e.g. drug abuse or medication) or a general medical condition (e.g. hyperthyroidism) and does not occur exclusively during a mood or psychotic disorder or a pervasive developmental disorder

to Alexander's terminology) (Alexander, 1930), or alien symptoms that are not normally experienced (egodystonic). If they are egosyntonic, it is more appropriate to use the diagnosis of anxious personality disorder, and if egodystonic, the diagnosis of GAD can be entertained.

ANXIETY, DEPRESSION, EATING AND PERSONALITY DISORDERS

All the disorders described in the classification system above are from the neurotic and stress-related disorders section of the two major classifications of mental disorder. Although these are linked to anxiety, they are not the only ones which are connected and depression, eating disorders and personality disorders are all linked in various ways to anxiety as outlined in Fig. 9.1 later in this book.

Depression is universally associated with anxiety, yet only one little diagnosis, mixed anxiety and depressive disorder (F41.2 in ICD-10) is acknowledged in the formal classification. This is a "subsyndromal" condition that is not really a diagnosis at all, and if either the anxiety or the depressive disorder reaches syndromal status (i.e. qualifies for a diagnosis elsewhere in the anxiety or depressive classification), the mixed diagnosis is abandoned. The evidence in clinical and research practice is very different:

- the correlation between anxiety and depressive symptoms is persistently high (around +0.7) (Tyrer, 1992a)
- diagnoses frequently change from anxiety to depression and vice versa during the course of the disorder (Kendell, 1974)
- "Pure" diagnoses are very rare; combined diagnoses of several disorders are more common (Ball *et al.*, 1995)
- Mixed anxiety–depressive disorders are the most common of all these conditions (Meltzer *et al.*, 1994).

This strong relationship suggests that neither anxiety nor depressive symptoms are useful diagnostic groupings and that they serve to indicate some underlying common conditions that manifest both sets of symptoms.

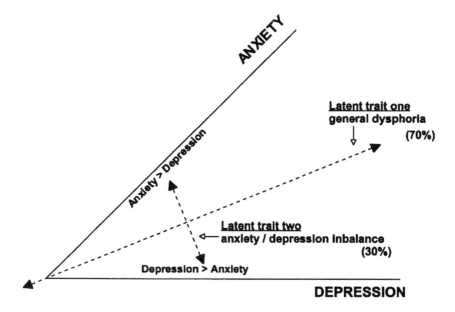

Fig. 5.2 The two latent traits for anxiety and depression. Reproduced from Goldberg and Huxley, 1992 (by permission of Tavistock/Routledge and the authors).

One elegant way of demonstrating this is to use latent trait analysis (Rasch, 1960). This was originally developed as a way of assessing the attainments of Danish school-children but has now been widely used in psychiatry to identify disorders that are not manifest on the surface (i.e. are latent) but which give rise to symptoms or disorders that can be measured. The latent trait model estimates the relationship of sets of symptoms to an underlying illness.

Goldberg and his colleagues (1987) have used latent trait analyses to determine the relationship between anxiety and depression and found that two dimensions, one predominantly of anxiety, and the other of depression, provided the best fit of symptoms of patients attending primary care with common psychiatric disorders (mainly anxiety and depressive ones). The two latent traits underlying the strong relationship between anxiety and depressive symptoms (correlation of 0.70 in this population) are illustrated in Fig. 5.2. The first trait (general dysphoria) represents the severity of the underlying disorder and the second latent trait as described as the anxiety/depression imbalance trait. This demonstrates that in some people with the underlying disorder, the symptoms are predominantly those of anxiety, whereas in others they are predominantly those of depression.

Although this is an interesting way of conceptualising the relationship between anxiety and depression, it does not provide an easy and straightforward way of classifying such individuals. The key feature appears to be vulnerability, i.e. the tendency of some individuals to respond to adversity by developing greater or lesser degrees of anxiety and depression and its counterpart, resilience, which protects against the development of such symptoms (Goldberg and Huxley, 1992).

Eating disorders are not anxiety ones but they deserve mention in this context. Anxiety is an early symptom in the development of both anorexia nervosa and bulimia (Hodes, 1993) and, while it is by no means certain that identification of the cause of the anxiety at this stage will prevent the onset of disorder, there is a great deal of evidence that different forms of secondary prevention (i.e. exploration and appropriate treatment to prevent progression of a disorder) can be particularly helpful in anxiety (Tyrer, 1994).

Personality disorder is not only in a different section of the psychiatric classification in ICD-10 but constitutes a different axis in DSM-IV (Axis I is mental disorders, Axis II is personality disorder). Wherever personality is placed, it is still closely connected to anxiety. The main classifications of personality disorder divide the disorders into three main groups or clusters. Cluster A, the odd or eccentric cluster, includes paranoid and schizoid personality disorders; Cluster B, the flamboyant or dramatic cluster, includes antisocial, histrionic, narcissistic, borderline and impulsive disorders; and Cluster C, the anxious-fearful cluster, includes dependent, anxious (ICD-10), avoidant (DSM-IV) and obsessive-compulsive (DSM-IV) and anankastic (ICD-10) personality disorders. Patients with obsessional symptoms are sometimes placed in a group on their own (Tyrer and Alexander, 1979; Cloninger, 1987) but still show important links to anxiety.

It is the last cluster that is so closely linked to anxiety (Lazare et al., 1966; Flick et al., 1993; Tyrer, 1985; Tyrer et al., 1997a) and it is fair to add that the connection was established much earlier in psychoanalysis

(Fromm, 1942). The notion of the anxious fearful personality lying at the heart of anxiety symptoms is an attractive hypothesis and there is a great deal to support it. The offensive word "neurotic", when used as a noun, describes a chronically anxious individual who may have depression, hypochondriasis, panic, and phobias at different times. The person ceases to have another identity once labelled "a neurotic" and this explains why the term is offensive. However, the fact that it does tend to be used repeatedly suggests that the problems it describes have diagnostic stability and persist. Avoidant personality disorder in DSM-IV (the ICD-10 equivalent, anxious personality disorder is very similar) describes a chronic fearful individual who avoids a wide range of situations to achieve protection from anticipated stress and, as a consequence, develops an increasingly restricted life style. This is closely linked to anxiety disorders in general and to social phobia in particular, for reasons that are not very clear and seem to be related to poor definitions as much as diagnostic overlap (see Chapter 9). Whenever anxiety appears to be an integral part of a person's existence, it is reasonable to search for a personality component.

IS THE CLASSIFICATION OF ANXIETY USEFUL?

I am sorry this has been such a turgid chapter; most discussions about classification in psychiatry are. It gives a glimpse of some of the difficulties of formalising the description of the anxiety disorders, which has its successes and failures. Its success is in identifying a number of important fundamentals in the main classification; the separation of unfocused from situational anxiety, the identification of disorders precipitated by internal and external stimuli, and the extremely valuable splitting of stress-related adjustment disorders from mainstream anxiety ones. These may not appear that exciting, but they assume greater importance when treating anxiety.

The failures are many. The conspicuous absence of all attempts to link anxiety and depression except in the underhand way of combining them subsyndromally, is a blot on the diagnostic landscape which no amount of argument can remove. It is for this reason mainly why I consider the classification to have been a failure (Tyrer, 1990). Instead of seeing the broad picture and getting it right, far too much attention has been paid in recent years to eternally dividing and subdividing the individual categories in a way that adds little to clinical practice. The real price of this failure is shown in Chapter 9 of this book; the issue of comorbidity is a direct consequence of our failure to divide anxiety at its proper joints; instead, we have been breaking up the bones and desperately trying to fit them together again. The sad outcome of this is that Osler's description at the beginning of this chapter is a better brief classification of anxiety disorders than anything that follows.

Chapter 6

DRUG TREATMENT OF ANXIETY

There are two standard ways of describing treatments for a range of disorders; the treatments can be listed and their applications to various disorders discussed, or the disorders described separately together with their individual treatments. As might be expected from the previous chapter, I have chosen the first approach, mainly because the clarity in the description of treatments is much better than that in the description of disorders. However, before describing the individual drugs, it is necessary to discuss the general principles of drug treatment with particular reference to the treatment of anxiety. The following text is written on the assumption that the reader knows very little about basic pharmacological terms and I apologise to the more experienced readers who will find some of my explanations unnecessary.

DRUGS AS SYMPTOMS SUPPRESSANTS

The word "cure" has been used in the past far too frequently in the treatment of all disorders, not just psychiatric ones. A treatment can only be regarded as a cure if it produces a fundamental and permanent change in the course of a disease which eradicates it from the body. The same can apply to a symptom or behaviour as much as a disease. Examples of cures are the treatment of an infection by an antibiotic (to which the infecting organism is sensitive) and the treatment of pernicious anaemia with vitamin B12 injections (which only remains a cure if the injections continue to be administered).

Of course, many treatments may appear to be cures if they are administered just before the disorder is set to resolve spontaneously.

Thirty-six years ago I was involved in a Cambridge University expedition collecting herbal remedies from native witch doctors (ngangas) in Central Africa. Among the many conditions treated by these remedies, one appeared five times more often than any other; syphilis. This is because each of the stages of syphilis is followed by an apparent cure. The symptoms improve and disappear altogether but the organism has merely gone into hibernation and will reappear some years later unless the specific antibiotic for exterminating syphilis, penicillin, is administered. Those forms of anxiety, particularly adjustment reactions, which have a good outcome almost irrespective of treatment will therefore appear to be cured by any agent given at the time of maximum symptomatology.

Unlike many other symptoms in psychiatry, anxiety fluctuates dramatically from day to day and during the course of the day (see Fig. 2.10). If drugs merely suppress symptoms while they are present,

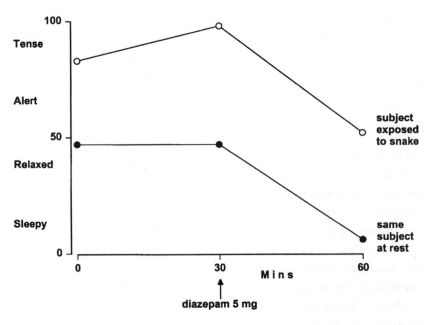

Fig. 6.1 Anti-anxiety drugs suppress symptoms of anxiety and produce sedation in non-anxious subjects.

they are likely to have different effects when the symptoms are absent. This view is supported by the anxiety ratings of a person who received an anti-anxiety drug, diazepam, on one occasion when very anxious (after being exposed to a snake in a laboratory test) and on another received the same drug in the same dosage while sitting at rest.

The results showed that when anxious the drug was effective in removing anxiety, but when anxiety was absent the drug merely created the adverse effect of sedation. A drug which genuinely corrected an abnormality in the body's function would not show such a generalised "blunderbuss" effect as does diazepam here.

Another consequence of this general rule is that when patients stop taking an anti-anxiety drug, their symptoms will return if the disorder has not naturally resolved during the course of the drug treatment. In technical terms this is described as *relapse,* but it is more accurate to describe it as a *return* of symptoms, particularly if they are very similar to the symptoms that existed before the drug treatment began. This issue is particularly important when discussing problems following the discontinuation of drug treatment, when withdrawal symptoms in drugs that promote addiction also complicate the picture.

THE DEGREE OF SEDATION PRODUCED BY A DRUG IS RELATED TO THE INTENSITY OF ANXIETY

Not all anti-anxiety drugs are sedatives but most have some calming action that can result in sedation. In Fig. 6.2, we see the Yerkes-Dodson curve again. In the first part of the figure, a sedative drug is given at a time of extreme anxiety (time 1) when symptoms are intense and function is beginning to disintegrate. The drug, if effective, will move the person back down the Yerkes-Dodson curve so that they are functioning more effectively and have only moderate anxiety symptoms. At this time, one hour later, the subject will almost certainly feel much better and have no symptoms of sedation. At time 2 however, the anxiety symptoms are only of moderate intensity and so administration of the drug will move the subject down the Yerkes-Dodson curve to a point of low anxiety in which performance is reduced. Sedation is much more common under

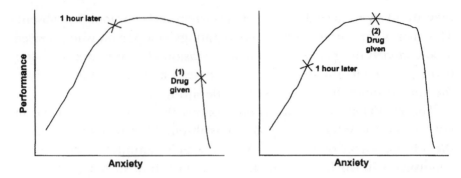

Fig. 6.2 Sedation depends on when the drug is given in the Yerkes-Dodson curve.

these circumstances and also explains the (at first unusual) findings shown in Fig. 6.1.

With the information we have already derived illustrating that anxiety changes greatly from day to day, it is important that the time of administration of any drug has some connection to the symptoms experienced. For this reason, many sedative anxiety drugs are prescribed in what is commonly called a prn basis, which is a common abbreviation for *pro re nata* (as the time arises).

Nevertheless, the phenomenon of tolerance — the tendency for drug effects to become less with repeated dosage — also has to be taken into account when predicting the sedative effect of a drug, and this is discussed later with particular reference to the benzodiazepines.

ANXIETY AND DEPRESSION

Despite all the psychological influences pulling anxiety and depression in opposite directions, we have found out in the previous chapter that they are common bedfellows and cannot stop being intimate with each other. This can be quite a problem when prescribing any form of treatment, though particularly with drugs. Depression with anxiety is often called agitated depression and depression without anxiety is (or in which the depression is much stronger than the presence of any anxiety symptoms) often called retarded depression (although both these terms have become less used in recent years). However, in both cases the presence of depression tends to reduce anxiety symptoms somewhat because depression reduces the speed of bodily and mental functions. Indeed, many people have drawn attention to the similarities between depression and hibernation in animals.

If a person has significant degrees of both anxiety and depression, a sedative anti-anxiety drug may merely remove the anxiety, bringing depression to the fore and making the patient feel much worse.

This close relationship is shown in Fig. 6.3, in which the relationship between anxiety and depression over a 12-year period is illustrated. The patient concerned had a mixed anxiety-depressive diagnosis

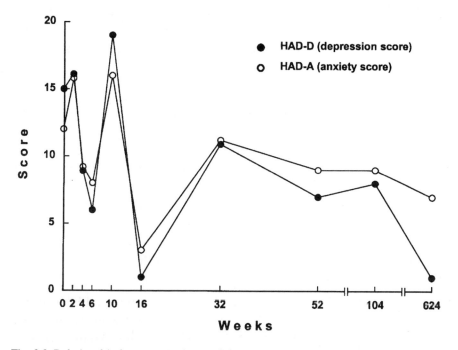

Fig. 6.3 Relationship between anxiety and depressive symptoms in a woman presenting at the age of 20 with generalised anxiety and followed up for 12 years. The ratings are from the Hospital Anxiety and Depression Scale (Zigmond and Snaith, 1983) which has depression scores (HAD-D) and anxiety scores (HAD-A) ranging between 0 and 21. (Reproduced with permission from Helen and Nicholas Seivewright in connection with the Nottingham Study of Neurotic Disorder.)

(i.e. qualified for the diagnoses of both dysthymic (chronic depressive) disorder and generalised anxiety disorder and also had a personality disorder. The correlation (r) between self-rated anxiety and depressive symptoms using the Hospital Anxiety and Depression Rating Scale (HADS) (which has both anxiety (HADS-A) and depression (HADS-D) components) (Zigmond and Snaith, 1983) is 0.95 for this patient. Whilst agreements between anxiety and depressive symptoms are normally a little lower than this (around 0.7), the close affinity between them cannot be cast aside as an artefact or an error; it is worthwhile reflecting on this when we consider that depression is not classified with the anxiety disorders and is in a completely different section of the classification (mood disorders) in both major classifications.

We will learn later that anti-depressive drugs are as effective as conventional anti-anxiety agents when given over a long period, and if depression is a prominent feature with the anxiety, it is understandable that this may influence the choice of treatment.

MARKED PLACEBO EFFECTS IN ANXIETY

Take a look in the window of your nearest shop selling herbal remedies. "Change from being tired and exhausted to feeling terrific and full of energy with Supernova , the new drug extract from galactic bark". "Nervous, can't concentrate, can't sleep; what you need is Naturecalm, the new natural way of restoring you to healthy balance". "Panicky, can't relax, can't concentrate — R-r-r-relax in a bath of lavasalts, nature's way of calming down when the volcano has erupted".

Are all these claims bogus and, if so, why do so many people believe them? In most countries people spend their own money buying these remedies, often in large quantities, and in those countries in which they are available through the state, such as France, the health budget is creaking under the strain.

The main reason is probably the placebo effect. I add the word "probably" because there is just the off-chance that one or more of these remedies is indeed a major new advance in the treatment of anxiety which is, as yet, undiscovered because the cost of carrying out the investigations necessary to prove its effectiveness cannot be supported by the small countries concerned. Placebo means "I will please" in Latin and describes the tendency for all remedies to have a non-specific beneficial effect when first administered and which wears off after a few weeks in most cases.

In randomised controlled trials, the commonest way of evaluating the effectiveness of drug treatment in any disorder, initial comparisons have to be made with placebo tablets or "dummy pills", which look exactly the same as the active tablets and therefore neither investigator nor patient know which is the active one (so called "double-blind" procedure. Even if the active drug is markedly superior to the placebo tablets, to begin with they appear very similar and it is only after 2–3 weeks, when the "placebo effects" are wearing off that significant advantages have been shown by the active drug.

There are several reasons for this. Firstly, when people invest in any form of treatment they want to make it work and, initially at any rate, convince themselves it is working. Psychologists call this phenomenon "cognitive dissonance"; once the decision has been made (to buy a herbal remedy, to take part in a clinical trial knowing you may receive dummy tablets) you want to justify your choice by feeling better. Disillusionment only sets in some time later when the effects wear off but, even then, people may still argue that the dummy pill is working because it did at first and therefore it needs to be given in higher dosage or more frequently to show its main effects. Secondly, dummy pills have no side effects and so whatever else happens, the person is unlikely to have any serious new symptoms from taking the pills. (Even this cannot be discounted absolutely; we will read later about the nocebo effect [from the Latin "I will harm"] which can reveal very unpleasant side effects from dummy pills).

The third reason is that when people take placebo tablets (or placebo injections), they stimulate the natural substances in the blood that remove pain and promote calm and satisfaction. These substances, termed endorphins, are related to the opiates such as heroin and morphine but are internally produced by the body to counteract pain and distress. The fact that a dummy pill can stimulate the release of endorphins shows the power of the psyche; it is not the pill that releases the endorphins but the belief that the pill is working.

ANTI-ANXIETY DRUGS ARE POTENTIALLY ADDICTIVE

This statement may surprise some people. Why should a treatment for anxiety which is only designed to remove the anxiety, be regarded in the same way as heroin, cocaine and similar drugs? In principle I agree with this objection, but it is an unfortunate fact, and painful experience for many people, that almost every new breakthrough in the drug treatment of anxiety has begun with tremendous optimism and excitement but has ended sooner or later, in disgrace or despair because of the addictive problems it has created.

Opium, morphine, cocaine, chloral, barbiturates, benzodiazepines — the list continues to grow and yet the drug industry and clinicians still fall for the latest new compound that "has not shown any signs of dependence in preliminary studies". If doctors behaved as though all these drugs were addictive right from the beginning, many of the problems created would have been avoided. It is therefore wise to be sceptical and cautious when reading these claims.

It is as well to be aware of these general principles when discussing each of the major compounds that have been used in the treatment of anxiety and which continue to be developed using much more vigorous methodology than in the past. The drug groups will be discussed in the order of their importance (which usually correlates with their volumes of prescription) and the ones licensed for the treatment of anxiety will be discussed before those that are not.

DRUGS USED FOR THE TREATMENT OF ANXIETY

The main drugs used for treating anxiety are shown in Table 6.2. The fact they are used for this purpose does not mean they are necessarily licensed for treatment. In clinical practice, this need not be of concern provided that proper justification is given for treatment outside the licensed indications.

Table 6.1 Principles of Drug Treatment in Anxiety

Drug treatment suppresses symptoms; it does not cure anxiety

The degree of sedation produced by a drug is related to the intensity of anxiety

Anxiety is rarely separate from depression and this may affect choice of drug treatment

Placebo effects are more marked in anxiety than almost any other mental disorder

All new drug treatments of anxiety should be regarded as addictive until proved otherwise

Table 6.2 Classification of Anti-anxiety Drugs

Drug Group	Common Members of Group	Main Mechanism of Action
Sedative/hypnotic	(main group): benzodiazepines (subsidiary groups): (a) barbiturates (b) cyclopyrrolones (c) propanediols (d) miscellaneous	Facilitation of γ-aminobutyric acid (GABA) transmission
Azospirodecanediones	buspirone	Partial agonists of 5-HT$_1$ receptors
Beta-blocking drugs	propranolol	Peripheral beta-blockade
Antihistamines	promethazine chlorpheniramine	Histamine-receptor blockade
Antipsychotic drugs	chlorpromazine, flupenthixol	
Tricyclic antidepressants	amitriptyline, dothiepin, trimipramine, clomipramine, lofepramine	
Monoamine oxidase inhibitors (MAOIs)	phenelzine, moclobemide	
Serotonin re-uptake inhibitors (SSRIs)	fluoxetine, paroxetine	Probably linked to changes in noradrenergic and 5-HT receptors after regular treatment for three of more weeks. Short term relief of anxiety may also be noticed immediately with the more sedative tricyclic antidepressants

BENZODIAZEPINES

Benzodiazepines are (still) the most commonly prescribed psychotropic drugs in the world and are one of the few polysyllabic drug groups known to almost everybody. Part of this high profile is related to their problems rather than their assets. Benzodiazepines were discovered in the late 1930s but not investigated as drugs to treat mental health problems until the 1950s. They were introduced at a time when there were few satisfactory drugs available for anxiety and they rapidly became "wonder drugs" (in retrospect, this was quite a good phrase as now we often wonder how we could have been so stupid as to give them this label) and were promoted heavily.

The reason why benzodiazepines were so much better than the drugs which had come before is that they acted in a novel way in the nervous system. They are similar to other sedative-hypnotic drugs in action in that they stimulate activity in one of the most important neurotransmitters, γ-aminobutyric acid (GABA for short) which has general inhibitory effects. When GABA systems are activated, there is a general reduction of nerve cell activity. Benzodiazepines differ from other sedative-hypnotic drugs in that they also have special places where they act in the nervous system called benzodiazepine receptors. As we have described in Chapter 2, the receptor is a useful concept to describe how a drug will work in one setting but not in another. Like a lock, which will only respond to the action of a key which fits the lock exactly, a drug will only act on a receptor when it too fits, or binds to, the receptor exactly. In fact, the benzodiazepine receptor is not as precise a selector of keys as many other receptors in the nervous system and drugs which are not benzodiazepines but which are similar to them, can bind to these receptors, and so affect brain cell activity.

The ability of benzodiazepines to bind to the benzodiazepine receptors allows them to have a special influence on the cells possessing GABA receptors which is denied to other drugs. This means that they act at lower doses and are generally much safer that other compounds such as alcohol and barbiturates (Table 6.3). However, when benzodiazepines are withdrawn after regular long-term use, there can be problems which are directly linked to their GABA links; we will come to this later.

Table 6.3 Summary of Risks and Benefits of Benzodiazepines Compared with Other Anti-anxiety Drugs

Benefits	Risks
Quick-acting	Sensorimotor impairment
Wide safety margin	Pharmacological dependence
Liked by patients	Anterograde amnesia

CLINICAL USE

The benzodiazepines in clinical practice are listed in Table 6.4 together with their main clinical indications. The list used to be longer, because it was so profitable to market a benzodiazepine in the 1970s many unnecessary additions were added to the list (Tyrer, 1974). Despite the differences listed in Table 6.3 there is much more that is common than is different between benzodiazepines and if the list was reduced to three — diazepam, temazepam and clonazepam — all important clinical needs would be met.

The main uses of benzodiazepines are the treatment of anxiety and insomnia; as part of the programme for detoxifying patients from alcohol and other drugs; the treatment (and prevention) of epilepsy; and in the emergency treatment of seriously disturbed or aggressive behaviour. Only the first of these issues concerns us here, and this constitutes their major use. Before going into these in more detail, we need to be aware of the problems of dependence and how they influence the recommended use of these drugs.

BENZODIAZEPINE DEPENDENCE

Unlike most other forms of drug dependence, which involve illicit drugs or alcohol, benzodiazepine dependence involves prescribed drugs which lead to dependence by accident. In fact, for many years

Table 6.4 The Main Benzodiazepines Used in Clinical Practice

Drug (Trade name)	Available on NHS prescription	Normal daily dosage (mg)	Speed of action	Type of drug	Main clinical use
triazolam (Halcion)[+]	No	0.125–5	fast	short-acting	insomnia
lormetazepam	Yes	0.5–1.5	fast	short-acting	insomnia
alprazolam (Xanax)[+]	No	0.75–4	medium	short-acting	panic
loprazolam (Dormonoct)	Yes	1–2	fast	short-acting	insomnia
lorazepam (Ativan)	Yes	1–5	fast	short-acting	anxiety
clonazepam (Rivotril)	Yes	1.5–10	medium	long-acting	epilepsy*
diazepam (Valium)	Yes	4–30	fast	short-acting (but long-acting in chronic dosage)	anxiety epilepsy muscle spasm
nitrazepam (Mogadon)	Yes	5–15	medium	long-acting	insomnia
clobazam (Frisium)	Yes	10–30	fast	long-acting	epilepsy*
temazepam (Normison)	Yes	10–30	fast	short-acting	insomnia
chlordiazepoxide (Librium)	Yes	10–60	medium	long-acting	Anxiety and alcohol withdrawal
oxazepam (Serenid)	Yes	30–90	medium	short-acting	anxiety

* only used for epilepsy on NHS prescription
[+] not available in UK except on private prescription

(1960–1978) it was felt that benzodiazepines did not create dependence and the apparently excessive use of the drugs was an indication of their effectiveness, particularly in the treatment of anxiety, which was often "chronic". Although concern was expressed that too often medication was being prescribed for personal problems rather than real illness (Trethowan, 1975), real concern that dependence might be a significant problem with these compounds did not arise until 1980 (Committee on Review of Medicines, 1980; Tyrer, 1980). The change occurred when it was realised that a great number of people with persistent symptoms of anxiety were probably having withdrawal symptoms independent of their original anxiety disorder. These symptoms, together with the phenomenon of tolerance, constitute most of benzodiazepine dependence. Tolerance, the phenomenon of reduced drug effects with repeated use, is prominent after benzodiazepines in acute dosage but not usually a serious problem in long-term dosage for anxiety and sleep disorders. Someone who slept well on 5 mg of nitrazepam (Mogadon) in 1980 often sleeps just as well on the same dose now.

Those who have withdrawal symptoms as the main part of their what is now described as *low dose dependence* continue on their drugs unnecessarily for long periods. Approximately one in three of all patients prescribed benzodiazepines for longer than two months, are likely to develop a significant degree of dependence inasmuch as they are unable to stop the drug after an appropriate period of time because of withdrawal symptoms (Tyrer, 1986). It is worth stressing that this figure is much less than the popular press would have us imagine. This is probably because benzodiazepine dependence had such a high profile in the media that there has been a strong negative perception created about benzodiazepines which in some quarters has implied that they are "worse than heroin". This is an example of the "nocebo effect" (i.e. I will harm), the opposite of the placebo effect, which exaggerates the identification of dependence so that even if the dosage of medication does not change people, can still develop apparent (pseudowithdrawal) symptoms (Tyrer *et al.*, 1983; Tyrer, 1991).

Ideally, if we were able to identify who would become dependent on benzodiazepines, we could have no concern about the majority who would not develop benzodiazepine dependence. There are several factors predisposing towards dependence, including the choice of benzodiazepine, dosage of drug, duration of treatment and personality status of the patient.

There is evidence, but none is definitely conclusive, that short-acting (those which have a duration of action of 10 hours or less) and high potency benzodiazepines (those which only need to be given in low dosage, to produce the same effect as other benzodiazepines given in higher dosage) are more likely to induce dependence. Of the major benzodiazepines in clinical use listed in Table 6.4, triazolam (Halcion), alprazolam (Xanax) and lorazepam (Ativan), all potent benzodiazepines with relatively short half-lives, have been associated with many more problems with dependence than the other compounds. (Triazolam is now no longer available on NHS prescription).

The dosage and duration of drug treatment, as might be expected, also affects dependence, with higher dosage being more likely to induce dependence problems, but not to a great degree (Holton et al., 1992) and those with longer duration of treatment having greater problems in stopping treatment, but only up to one year of continuous treatment, not beyond (Holton and Tyrer, 1990; Holton, 1992). Unfortunately, these are statistical associations only and, as withdrawal problems can be established as early as four to six weeks of treatment (Fontaine et al., 1984; Power et al., 1985; Tyrer and Murphy, 1987), this is normally taken as the higher level of acceptable treatment duration.

The personality status of patients and dependence risk of benzodiazepines is an emotive subject. In our personal work we have found consistently that people with dependent and anxious personalities are more likely to develop withdrawal symptoms when they stop benzodiazepines (Tyrer et al., 1983; Murphy and Tyrer, 1991). This suggests that it is patients, rather than doctors or drugs, that are key to the development of dependence; but this is not a popular message. "Only wimps become tranquilliser junkies" was how one tabloid newspaper reported this finding after publication, and it was promptly followed by a formal complaint from self-help tranquilliser groups who objected to its implications. The word "only" is unfair, but the general gist of the message is correct (after making allowance for the vulgarity of expression).

To make the diagnosis of the benzodiazepine withdrawal syndrome, the following are necessary:

(a) symptoms must always follow drug reduction or withdrawal (usually within 5 days),
(b) there may be an increase in the previous symptoms of anxiety and/ or emergence of new symptoms that have not been experienced before, and
(c) some improvement should occur after the first 14 days of reduction.

The common symptoms of the benzodiazepine withdrawal syndrome are those of anxiety (palpitations, tingling, sweating, difficulty in concentration, irritability, tremor); hypersensitivity to sensory stimuli of all kinds (tinnitus, blurring of vision, formication (feeling of things crawling on the skin)); and (much less common) neurological symptoms such as epilepsy, paranoid psychotic symptoms and muscular twitching. These can almost be predicted from knowledge of the actions of benzodiazepines. They are all rebound effects that are the opposite of anxiety reduction, sedation and anticonvulsant effects. These can be predicted from the effects of benzodiazepines on GABA transmission and exactly the same symptoms can be created by giving a GABA antagonist (e.g. picrotoxin), suggesting that dependence problems can be described in terms of GABA stimulation (Cowen and Nutt, 1982).

It is also relevant that anxiety and insomnia in psychiatric patients can act as reinforcers in their own right for continued consumption of benzodiazepines and this is accentuated in those who abuse alcohol or take other sedative drugs (Griffiths and Weerts, 1997). This acts quite independently of withdrawal problems, fuelling continued consumption of drugs.

The adverse effects of benzodiazepines include addictive effects with alcohol and other depressant drugs, particularly other drugs of the sedative-hypnotic type, as would be predicted from Table 6.3. A major indication of excessive dosage is drowsiness. Anterograde amnesia (i.e. amnesia from the time of onset of drug action) may also be a problem in higher dosages, although it may have a beneficial effect in some conditions (e.g. premedication for dental phobia). All benzodiazepines (and all other sedative drugs) have a risk of psychomotor impairment. This is of special relevance when carrying out tasks that need co-ordination and vigilance (e.g. driving, monitoring machinery). Because anxiety fluctuates considerably from hour to hour, unwanted effects such as psychomotor impairment may be noted after acute anxiety has passed but the effects of the drug persist.

It is also important to note that benzodiazepines are well liked by patients. This can be considered as a handicap, as it is equally possible to argue that such liking constitutes a euphoriant effect of the drug that makes it prone to abuse (Griffiths and Weerts, 1997). However, if two classes of drug are equally efficacious at treating a problem, the one that is preferred by patients will normally be prescribed, mainly because compliance is such an important part of the treatment procedure.

OTHER SEDATIVES AND HYPNOTICS

As indicated in Table 6.2, the benzodiazepines are only one of the sedative-hypnotic group of drugs, all so-called because in therapeutic dosage (usually towards the upper end) they produce sedation and induce sleep. They share many characteristics with the benzodiazepines in that they act on the same neurotransmitter system, GABA. These drugs included chlormethiazole (Hemenevrin), the barbiturates (which nowadays should never be prescribed for anxiety and therefore are listed only for historical reasons), glutethimide (Doriden) (which has significant dependence potential), compounds containing chloral hydrate or similar salts (e.g. Noctec, Triclofos) and meprobamate (Equanil). In general, these drugs are not quite as effective as the benzodiazepines but still carry the same risk of dependence because they act in roughly similar ways. However, some of these, particularly the drugs containing chloral compounds still have a place, particularly in helping people to sleep. They are sufficiently different from the benzodiazepines for them to be used, sometimes as benzodiazepine substitutes, in helping to treat patients who are going through the withdrawal syndrome. However, they should not be used for more than a few weeks under these circumstances as they can cause dependence in their own right .

Two new drugs, zopiclone (Zimovane), a member of the cyclopyrrolone group of drugs, and zolpidem (Stilnoct) have also recently been introduced for the treatment of insomnia. They are not benzodiazepines but have somewhat similar actions and act on sites close to the main benzodiazepine receptor (Fig. 6.4). Although some

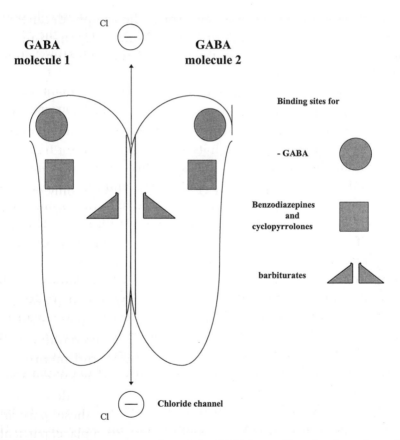

Fig. 6.4 The schematic representation of the GABA-benzodiazepine ionophore. Note that the ionophore has to have a negative charge (hence the chloride channel) and that the sites for GABA (χ-amino butyric acid), benzodiazepine and cyclopyrrolone binding are all relatively close.

advantages have been claimed for them over the benzodiazepines, particularly in terms of reduced dependence potential (which is rather stronger for zolpidem than zopiclone (Monti *et al.*, 1994; Rush and Griffiths, 1996), these remain to be confirmed as clinically advantageous and it is reasonable to regard these drugs as having equivalent risks of dependence as benzodiazepines.

BUSPIRONE

This drug is a member of a new group, the azospirodecanediones, which also includes compounds such as gepirone and ipsaperone, which might also become available for the treatment of anxiety or depression in the future.

Buspirone has one major advantage over the benzodiazepines; it does not produce dependence (Fontaine *et al.*, 1987; Lader, 1988), and so there is no reason in principle why it should not be continued for several months or even longer (although its main indication is for treatment of short- and medium term anxiety). Despite this obvious advantage, it has not proved to be a particularly popular drug and this appears to be a consequence of its major disadvantage; it is dysphoric, or more simply, it makes people feel bad. When this is combined with a short delay before its full effects are shown, it is easy to see why it has not become well established.

Buspirone, given in doses between 5 and 20 mg daily, is useful in the treatment of some patients with anxiety and is undoubtedly effective (Feighner *et al.*, 1982), although less effective than other drugs such as the benzodiazepines in more severe anxiety such as panic (Sheehan *et al.*, 1993). It has also been used to help people who are dependent on benzodiazepines with relative lack of efficacy (Ashton *et al.*, 1990).

Buspirone, despite failure to fulfil its potential, is still of interest because it acts, not on GABA receptors but on (serotonin) 5-HT_{1A} receptors. Increasingly, the importance of serotonin is becoming clear in both anxiety and depression (Eison, 1990) and it is likely that other azospirodecanediones may prove to be of more lasting value.

BETA-BLOCKING DRUGS, ANTIHISTAMINES AND OTHER ANTI-ANXIETY DRUGS

Beta-blocking drugs have been used for the treatment of some forms of anxiety from the time they were first reported as being of value in these disorders (Granville-Grossman and Turner, 1966; Tyrer and Lader, 1972) and now have an established place in clinical psychiatric practice (Birkett and Tyrer, 1990). This remains a relatively limited one; even though they are demonstrably more effective than placebo (Tyrer, 1992b), they are not effective in more severe forms of anxiety (Noyes et al., 1984; Birkett and Tyrer, 1990). It is likely that their major effects on the emotions are due to their peripheral effects (Eliasch et al., 1967; Bonn et al., 1972); peripheral and symptoms mediated through beta-receptors are most likely to be helped. These include awareness of fast heart beat, flushing, palpitations and tremor. The most obvious use of beta-blockers is in the treatment of performance anxiety in acute stress situations, such as speaking in public and playing a musical instrument. If avoidance of tremor is particularly important (e.g. playing the violin), beta-blocking drugs may be of particular help (James et al., 1977; 1983; James and Temple-Savage, 1984). Their efficacy in this regard gives some support to those theories of emotion that emphasise the peripheral aspects rather than the central one (e.g. the James-Lange theory) (Tyrer, 1973a). The main advantage of beta-blockers is that they have no sedative effects or sensorimotor impairment and have no risk of dependence.

Antihistamines are well established drugs with a long history of successful use in the treatment of mild anxiety and insomnia from childhood onwards. The sedative effects are rapid in onset but these overlap with drowsiness which can become a severe problem in daytime use. Although the dependence risk of these drugs is low, there is still some potential for abuse, with both cyclizine and diphenhydramine being reported as addictive. However, problems of withdrawal following long-term low dose treatment have not been reported.

ANTIPSYCHOTIC DRUGS

These drugs, ranging from the prototype chlorpromazine introduced in 1950 to the newer atypical drugs such as risperidone, clozapine, sertindole and olanzapine, are all effective in treating anxiety. They have not been subjected to rigorous comparison with other established drugs in recent years, but most older studies show them to be of roughly equivalent efficacy (Greenblatt and Shader, 1974; Young *et al.*, 1976), and they are still considered useful in clinical practice in a range of situations (Tyrer *et al.*, 1997b). There is also solid evidence confirming that they are of no risk with regard to dependence and, indeed, do not lead to tolerance of any serious degree (Aranko *et al.*, 1985). However, the main reason for caution is the danger that the irreversible syndrome of tardive dyskinesia might develop (Uhrbrand and Faurbye, 1960), and this confines their use to the short-term only, unless they are given for the treatment of anxiety in conjunction with psychotic disorders.

ANTIDEPRESSANTS

Although most antidepressants are not licensed for the treatment of anxiety (citalopram and paroxetine are exceptions), they have been used increasingly for this purpose since the furore over benzodiazepine dependence first began in the 1980s. This is not surprising, since from the mid-1960s, evidence had emerged that antidepressants were effective in the treatment of anxiety, even though, unlike the benzodiazepines, which helped immediately, their effects took between two and four weeks to develop adequately (Kahn *et al.*, 1986; Lipman *et al.*, 1986). This became prominent with the work of Klein mentioned in conjunction with panic in Chapter 5 (Klein, 1964, 1967, 1980). The fact that panic was not shown to be "pharmacologically dissected" by imipramine was not relevant; the evidence, begun with imipramine and extended to include monoamine oxidase inhibitors in the 1970s (Tyrer, 1973b; Tyrer *et al.*, 1973; Ravaris *et al.*, 1976), only served to blur the division between anxiety and depression that we, and others (Hudson and Pope, 1990), have found increasingly to be a shibboleth hardly worth retaining.

Because antidepressants were not considered to produce dependence, it was natural to change from sedative drugs with increasing problems associated with their use to well-tried "clean" antidepressants without such problems. This pressure became even stronger when the new class of antidepressants, the selective serotonin reuptake inhibitors (SSRIs), were introduced to a market saturated with antidepressants. These new antidepressants were of similar efficacy to the old ones in the treatment of depression (Kasper *et al.*, 1995), but were less likely to lead to suicide in overdose because they were less toxic (Cassidy and Henry, 1987; Farmer and Pinder, 1989; Montgomery *et al.*, 1992). When additional evidence came along that the SSRIs were possibly more effective in treating anxiety associated with depression than standard tricyclic antidepressants (Den Boer *et al.*, 1987; Dunbar *et al.*, 1991), an additional reason for choosing these drugs was found. The position now is that anxiety is regularly treated with antidepressants in all forms of clinical practice (Tyrer and Tyrer, 1993; Tyrer and Hallström, 1993) and the only variation is in the diagnostic choice for each compound or group.

In general, the SSRIs are more effective in obsessional disorders, in which clomipramine, despite being a tricyclic antidepressant, is also included as it has partial serotonin selection (Insel and Johar, 1987; Perse *et al.*, 1987); imipramine and other tricyclic antidepressants still vie with the SSRIs in the treatment of panic and generalised anxiety (Pollack *et al.*, 1994; Boulanger, 1995); and the SSRIs are now being investigated more in the treatment of phobias. The monoamine oxidase inhibitors, particularly the new reversible compounds that do not have the dietary restrictions associated with the old agents such as phenelzine and tranylcypromine, are now being targeted on social phobia. Preliminary evidence suggests that moclobemide, the main exemplar of the new compounds, is not as effective as phenelzine in treating social phobia, but is at least is better than placebo (Versiani *et al.*, 1992).

The curious reader will already have picked up one of the uses of the new diagnoses of anxiety disorders, the tagging of new drugs used to treat them. This is mainly a marketing ploy. A "hole" is discovered in the market in that there seems to be a need for a treatment for a certain condition, and if a new diagnosis is created, a hole is also created overnight. The enterprising pharmaceutical company decides that its new compound is nicely tailored to the new diagnosis and all the resources of the research team are concentrated on this condition. One of the rules of investigation is that the new compound must not be tested in comparison with other diagnostic groups, as these might reveal that it has no specific association with the diagnosis under study. After the end of the series of investigations, it is hoped the new compound will be better than placebo and at least as good as a reference drug from the same group. Further marketing then goes into operation to imply (never quite state directly) that the new drug has specific value in treating the new psychiarric disorder. The best example of this is alprazolam, a powerful benzodiazepine used for the treatment of panic disorder with agoraphobia. The drug and new diagnosis were introduced almost simultaneously to great acclaim and commercial success; no wonder my colleagues in the United States sometimes change the name of panic disorder and agoraphobia to the simple acronym, ADS, the alprazolam deficiency syndrome.

The only snag from the extension of the use of antidepressants to treat anxiety was the fourth principle governing the use of antianxiety drugs in Table 6.1, that all new drug treatments of anxiety should be regarded as addictive until proved otherwise. The problems of dependence are not just confined to the benzodiazepines; they occur to some extent with the antidepressants also. The subject has been known about for some time. Both monoamine oxidase inhibitors and tricyclic antidepressants are associated with problems of withdrawal, in some instances with the MAOIs having the greater problems (Tyrer, 1984; Dilsaver, 1994). However, the SSRIs have been particularly associated with unusual symptoms following withdrawal, including nausea, dizziness and other somatic symptoms (Haddad, 1997; Zajecka *et al.*, 1997) and as these seem to be more severe with the SSRIs of shorter duration of action (shorter half-life), such as paroxetine, and least in the SSRIs of longest half-life (fluoxetine), it shows embarrassingly close links to the controversy over short vs long half-life benzodiazepines in the precipitation of benzodiazepine dependence.

The sensitivity over this issue is such that the term "dependence", or even "withdrawal" is becoming outlawed in favour of the neutral phrase, discontinuation syndromes. Whatever it is called, the truth will out in time.

CHOICE OF DRUG TREATMENT IN ANXIETY

In choosing a drug treatment for anxiety, there are several issues which need to be addressed before the drug is chosen, the main one is the likely duration of treatment. If it is likely that the drug will only be needed for a short time (e.g. for an adjustment disorder), then it is likely that a benzodiazepine will be chosen unless the patient has a dependent personality or other characteristics predisposing to dependence. If, however, the event leading to the anxiety is of particular emotional significance for the patient, it would be wise not to give a benzodiazepine in high dosage in case anterograde amnesia (amnesia during the period of major drug action) developed and prevented subsequent adjustment to the event.

If the anxiety is likely to need longer term treatment, an antidepressant might be considered but as there is a delay in the onset of therapeutic effects, a benzodiazepine might be given for a short time (e.g. 2 weeks) simultaneously, on the clear understanding that this will not be repeated. Although the tricyclic antidepressants are now generally considered to be "dirty old drugs" in many quarters because of their many side effects, it is important to note that one of these side effects, sedation, can be very helpful to the anxious patient. The sedation, unlike the main anti-anxiety effects, begins immediately after administration of the drug, and so could take the place of a sedative-hypnotic drug during the first 20 days of therapy. Trimipramine (100–200 mg), dothiepin (75–150 mg) and amitriptyline (75–175 mg) are the main sedative antidepressants available and, if a benzodiazepine is being given simultaneously for the first few weeks, it may be more successfully withdrawn under cover of the antidepressant (Tyrer *et al.*, 1996).

If dependence is considered to be a major risk (e.g. in the treatment of alcohol withdrawal), then buspirone could be used in the longer term while the risks of epilepsy and other acute problems could be offset by prescribing a benzodiazepine such as chlordiazepoxide (20–100 mg daily) in steadily reducing dosage. Low dose neuroleptic drugs such as thioridazine (25–75 mg daily) and flupenthixol (0.5–1.5 mg daily) could also be considered if dependence is considered a long term risk.

Table 6.5 Comparison of the Issues Determining the Choice of an Anti-anxiety Drug

Drug group	Speed of action	Sedation and sensori-motor impairment	Risk of dependence	Efficacy	Main indications
Sedative/ hypnotics	Fast (< 2 hours)	Significant but dose-related	Relatively great in long-term treatment	Excellent	Time-limited - treatment (e.g. alcohol withdrawal)
Azospiro-decanediones	Fairly slow (2–5 days)	Very little	Very low	Good	Anxiety in abuse-prone situations (e.g. chronic alcohol abuse)
Antipsychotic drugs	Fairly slow	Little in low dosage	Very low	Fair	Anxiety in presence of psychotic symptoms
Antihistamines	Fast	Present to some degree	Slight	Fair	Mild anxiety and insomnia
Antidepressants - tricyclic	Slow (2–5 wks)	Variable, depending on dose and drug	Very low	Good	Persistent anxiety/panic associated with chronic insomnia
Antidepressants - SSRIs and reversible MAOIs	Slow (2–5 wks)	Very little	Low	Very good	Yet to be determined
Beta-blocking drugs	Fast	None	None	Good in some instances	Performance anxiety

The choice of an SSRI or an MAOI such as moclobemide, in place of a tricyclic antidepressant, may also be made. Clomipramine is a cheap compromise in this task; no studies have shown clomipramine (50–200 mg/day) to be less effective than a more respectable SSRI in the treatment of anxiety. The main problem will be when the treatment is considered to be over and "discontinuation problems" may arise. The additional provision of brief psychotherapy during the treatment may help to maintain progress after the antidepressant is withdrawn (Wiborg and Dahl, 1996).

The full choice is shown in Table 6.5. It is not always an easy one and it helps to consider all aspects of drug treatment, initial therapy, maintenance treatment, and effects of withdrawal, before the choice is made.

SUMMARY

Drugs are effective in anxiety but their correct use involves a judicious use of selecting the right compound, using it for the most appropriate time and anticipating, not merely reacting to, any problems. Combining drug and psychological treatments is also an excellent way of getting the best out of both of them. The exact diagnosis of the patient being treated is of lesser importance; do not let it get in the way of answering the other questions.

Chapter 7

PSYCHOLOGICAL TREATMENT OF ANXIETY

In a world in which psychiatric treatments were matched with disorders, it would be natural for psychological treatments to be the preferred treatments for anxiety. Unfortunately, for a number of reasons best explained by "levels" of disorder, almost all treatment modalities have a place in the management of anxiety (Tyrer and Steinberg, 1998). There are several reasons why one might expect psychological treatments, in addition to psychoanalytical approaches described earlier, might be helpful in overcoming anxious symptoms.

PSYCHOLOGICAL ORIGINS OF ANXIETY

Although there are some indications that an anxious temperament is genetically determined, it is also easy to see how anxiety can develop as a result of experiences. Thus the statement that anxiety in adult life can be generated by insecure attachments in childhood has obvious face validity. It also receives some support from other quarters. Much of this evidence derives from the attachment theory, a concept that was developed almost entirely from the work of John Bowlby who formulated its implications in one of his later works (Bowlby, 1973).

Primarily through the process of simple observation, Bowlby noted that good attachment is normally established through a relationship between an infant and mother in which warmth, intimacy and consistency are the key elements. Separation anxiety is demonstrated when the child is parted from its mother and is manifest by obvious distress such as crying and fearful responses which are usually separated into three phases: (i) protest, including crying and searching behaviour; (ii) despair, in which the child is apathetic and miserable; and (iii) detachment, in which the child appears to have "given up" on his or her maternal relationship and developed a kind of pseudo-independence in which apparent self-confidence hides underlying vulnerability. During development, the child learns to tolerate increasing degrees of maternal separation, but Bowlby postulated that attachment behaviour was never completely outgrown and that unresolved separation anxiety was associated with anxiety in adult life (with the stage of detachment being in danger of developing into antisocial personality disorder). Although this has never been assessed directly, there is good evidence that infants as young as six months differ in their responses to separation and that future anxiety temperament, if not anxiety symptoms, can be identified at this stage.

It is also well established that children learn from their parents and this includes "learned anxiety" in many instances. If a young child is with an agoraphobic mother for most of the day it is not difficult to see that, in time, the child will learn to avoid the same phobic situations and develop identical phobic fears. Bearing in mind that the major influences on a growing child are those provided by both parents, it is easy to see how maladaptive behaviour can develop in children also as a matter of course. It is therefore easy to postulate that a psychological treatment would be the best way of reversing this process in adult life.

The main psychological treatments available for anxiety are based on the notion that pathological anxiety in its many forms consists of maladaptive and inappropriate responses to stimuli which have been generated as much from past experience as constitition. These treatments are behaviour therapy, cognitive therapy and related techniques such as anxiety management training. There is also a range of alternative therapies which are less well researched but are worthy of mention, not least because anxiety disorders are extremely prone to the placebo effect.

BEHAVIOUR THERAPY

The best established psychological treatment for anxiety disorders is behaviour therapy for phobic disorders, particularly agoraphobia and simple phobias. Behaviour therapy is devised from learning theory and particularly from the two forms of conditioning pioneered by Pavlov and Skinner. Pavlovian conditioning is often described as classical conditioning but now has little application in the treatment of mental illness but is worth describing because of its primacy. Classical conditioning is illustrated by Pavlov's early experiments whereby dogs were conditioned to salivate at the sound of a bell. A hungry dog (and indeed a hungry human) salivates at the thought and approach of food (unconditioned stimulus), but if a bell is sounded just before the food is produced, it becomes a conditioned stimulus so that when the bell alone is sounded the animal will salivate in the anticipation of food.

The process of classical conditioning with Pavlov's dogs is illustrated in Fig. 7.1. It is only one of the many examples in daily life where unconditioned stimuli leading to unconditioned responses can be made into conditioned responses by linking the unconditioned stimulus to a conditioned one. The acquisition of a conditioned stimulus is more rapid when there is a short duration between the pairing of the conditioned stimulus and the unconditioned stimulus. In general, it has been found that if the conditioned stimulus precedes the unconditioned stimulus by around half a second, more rapid acquisition of the conditioned stimulus and response is made.

The term "extinction" is used to describe the gradual disappearance of a conditioned response and this occurs when the conditioned stimulus is repeatedly presented without the unconditioned one. Thus Pavlov demonstrated this in his dogs by repeatedly sounding the bell after the dogs had become conditioned but then not giving them food subsequently.

Another important concept deriving from conditioning is that of generalisation. This is the process whereby once the conditioned response has been established in connection with a given stimulus, that this same response can also be evoked by other stimuli that are similar to, but not exactly the same as, the original conditioned stimulus. Thus

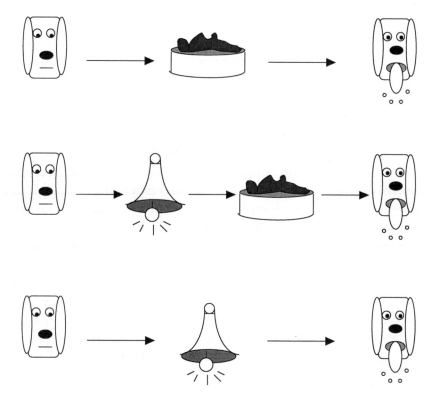

Fig. 7.1 Classical (Pavlovian) conditioning.

the sound of another instrument apart from a bell maybe just as effective in creating salivation than the original bell and this may quickly generalise to other similar noise stimuli subsequently. The opposite of generalisation is discrimination, whereby two stimuli can be sufficiently well distinguished to create a conditioned response for one but not for the other. Thus sounds of different pitch can be discriminated so that only one leads to a conditioned response.

Because most psychiatric symptoms and behaviour have many stimuli involved in their generation, there are now relatively few applications of classical conditioning in treatment. The main one is aversion therapy (attempting to associate a pleasant unconditioned stimulus with an unpleasant conditioned one so that the behaviour is altered). The ways in which this is being used in practice, as, for example, in the treatment of alcohol dependence by giving an emetic drug (to induce vomiting) immediately before drinking, have not been particularly successful and they are somewhat punitive in clinical practice.

Operant conditioning (sometimes called instrumental learning) adopts the alternative policy of using behaviour to change behaviour. This was popularised by Skinner (1938), an American psychologist, but most of its principles had been laid down earlier by Thorndike (1911). In this type of conditioning, behaviour becomes changed quite voluntarily, because its occurrence is reinforced by being rewarded. Both Thorndike and Skinner described experiments in which this could be tested and replicated. Thus, Thorndike places cats in puzzle boxes from which they could only escape and reach some food by unlocking the box, using a manoeuvre such as stepping on a pedal or pulling on a string. Because cats are curious and explore their immediate environment thoroughly, eventually the cat carries out the appropriate manoeuvre to allow the box to be opened and to reach the food. Subsequently, the time taken for the same cat to find the way out of the box becomes steadily shorter. This was the first example of what is now called trial-and-error learning. Eventually the cat becomes so conditioned that it can escape from the puzzle box immediately and obtain the food. These experiments led Thorndike to oppose a "law of effect" and stated that voluntary behaviour that is paired with reward is reinforced.

Skinner developed this further by introducing what is now commonly called the Skinner box. This usually involves the incorporation of a lever or set of buttons with a dish for food underneath it and a small light bulb above it. Every time an appropriate button is pecked or the right lever is pressed, a pellet of food is released into the food dish. Hungry pigeons placed in a Skinner box will peck at everything randomly but eventually peck the appropriate button which releases the pellet of food. This release of food is the conditioned response and will quickly become the preferred behaviour after repeated trials of the animal in the same box. This is demonstrated in Fig. 7.2.

The same principles of learning theory apply to operant as well as to classical conditioning. Thus if the pigeon is not rewarded when it pecks the appropriate button, the behaviour becomes steadily less frequent

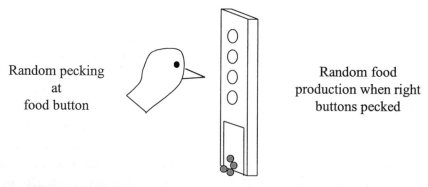

Random pecking
at
food button

Random food
production when right
buttons pecked

Unconditioned behaviour

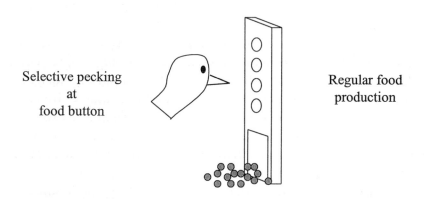

Selective pecking
at
food button

Regular food
production

Conditioned behaviour

Fig. 7.2 Operant (Skinnerian) conditioning.

and goes through the phenomenon of extinction. If the animal is then allowed to rest but then returns to the same box, it will tend to peck at the same buttons again despite the earlier process of extinction. This phenomenon, known as partial recovery, also occurs with classical conditioning.

Similarly, discrimination can also be demonstrated, for example by only releasing the pellet of food when a light is on in the box and the pecked but not when the button is pecked and the light is off. defined positive reinforcers as any stimulus which increased ᴜᵢᵤ ᵖability of the operant behaviour and a negative reinforcer which was aversive and reduced the incidence of the behaviour. In the animal studies, the most common positive reinforcer is food (and water) and the most common negative reinforcer is an electric shock.

There are different ways in which reinforcement can be introduced into operant conditioning. The common method is to use continuous reinforcement, which leads to a maximum response in which reinforcement takes place after every conditioned response. However, in partial reinforcement only some of the conditioned responses are being reinforced and this can be modified into giving the reward at fixed or variable intervals or sometimes after fixed or variable ratios of responses (e.g. food is delivered once after five pecks have been made at the button).

The main behavioural treatment for phobias is exposure therapy. Although this has been known for a long time, it has only recently been formulated in practice. Those who have seen the Alfred Hitchcock film *Vertigo* will see a classical example of it (training to get used to heights) before it was ever part of standard therapy. The core principle of exposure is "persuasion of the sufferer to repeatedly confront the cues that evoke fear and panic until the distress habituates" (Marks and Marks, 1990, p. 294). In learning terms, exposure therapy regards the phobia (unreasonable fear) and subsequent avoidance of the phobic stimulus as a maladaptive conditioned behaviour that needs to be extinguished. This is best achieved by deconditioning the maladaptive behaviour patterns and counter-conditioning them with better adaptive ones. This is illustrated in Fig. 7.3 which shows how the maladaptive pathway of fear-avoidance — reinforcement of fear is counter-conditioned by exposure-reduced fear — more exposure.

The principles of exposure therapy are extremely straightforward; indeed, they were presented in almost their current therapeutic form by Charles Darwin in 1872. Despite this, the application of this approach in psychiatry has not been a particularly smooth one. The original form of exposure was desensitisation, and originally this was presented as desensitisation-in-imagination. The sufferer had to think about the

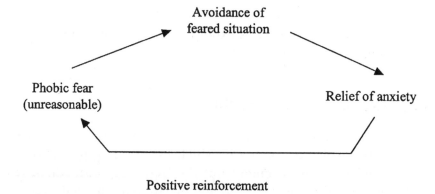

Maladaptive conditioning in the generation and persistence of phobias

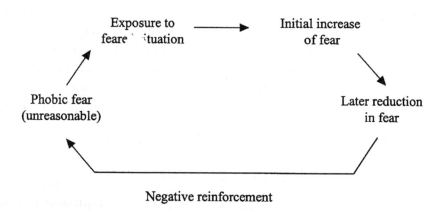

Fig. 7.3 Origin of agoraphobia and its treatment by exposure.

phobic stimulus when in a relaxed state and the intention was for the relaxation feeding to be paired with the phobic thinking so that it no longer evoked fear. The theory came from the work of a South African psychiatrist, Joseph Wolpe (1958) who introduced a theory of reciprocal inhibition derived from neurology, which postulated that it was necessary to present both the agonist (fearful) and antagonist (relaxation) stimuli together in order to get a learned association and thereby therapeutic improvement. In fact, many studies have shown that desensitisation-in-imagination is not as effective as exposure and there is really no place for it in behaviour therapy nowadays.

DIFFERENT FORMS OF EXPOSURE

Abundant research in the past 20 years has demonstrated that it is not the particular technique in which exposure is delivered that is the key issue in improvement but the frequency with which it is undertaken. At first it used to be thought that therapist-guided exposure would be much more effective than rough and ready exposure carried out by the phobic patient under their own effort. In fact, not only has it not found to be particularly helpful to have the therapist directly involved in exposing the patient, but training for exposure can be given equally well by computer with no direct contact with the therapist at all (Ghosh and Marks, 1987). If contact with the therapist is felt to be necessary, and some form of monitoring of progress is necessary at various points of treatment, then this should be reinforced by homework tasks to be carried out between sessions, so that exposure will continue to take place repeatedly with patients monitoring themselves (Mathews *et al.*, 1981).

EFFICACY OF EXPOSURE TREATMENT

The evidence that exposure therapy is effective in phobic disorders has now been shown in over 100 studies. This shows that, compared with almost all other treatments, exposure therapies are more effective in reducing phobic fear and avoidance (van Balkom *et al.*, 1997). It is also more effective than other psychological treatments in post-traumatic stress disorder (Foa *et al.*, 1991).

The type of phobia has relatively little impact on the success of treatment, although there is good evidence that phobias that are more clear cut and specific, such as most of the simple phobias (like fears of lightning, dogs, thunder, etc.) are more successfully treated than the more diffuse phobias of agoraphobia and social phobia. Unfortunately, the simple phobias are also the least handicapping and so the introduction of behaviour therapy has not had the effect predicted by the late Hans Eysenck, who predicted in 1975 "that within a generation, psychologists in mobile treatment trucks will travel round the country and eliminate phobias and other neurotic disorders entirely".

There is also an unfortunate fact that keeps intruding even though one cannot help being impressed by the high rate of recovery maintained by patients who have received behaviour therapy. This is that many patients either refuse to consider behaviour therapy or never complete an adequate programme of treatment. Bearing in mind that highly motivated, committed patients are more likely to do well than those who are unable to engage your complete therapy, it is reasonable to argue that these figures may not be representative of phobic patients as a whole.

A second troubling clinical experience also obtrudes on these fine figures; a significant proportion of phobic patients remain fearful despite repeatedly exposing themselves to their phobic stimuli on an almost daily basis. These people have been treating themselves with behaviour therapy for years, exactly as specified by the authorities in learning theory, yet have failed to make any progress. Why should this be so? One easy explanation is that there is something deficient in the way these people are practising their exposure and it is not reinforcing reduction in fear as Fig. 7.3 demonstrates. Unfortunately, this is unlikely to be the case in almost all instances. When the individuals come for treatment, even if they are persuaded that the approach that they have been trying for years is going to be successful in the hands of a trained therapist, they tend not to improve. One possibility is that symptoms of panic, known as the most severe type of anxiety, "unlearn" again during exposure and that if panic attacks are dealt with successfully in the course of treatment (e.g. by deep breathing and relaxation exercises, or sometimes by paradoxical stimulation, e.g. thinking of the most severe panic you have ever had in trying to make it happen) then this problem could be overcome. Sometimes it can, but more often it fails. Many individuals in this category do not come into the statistics for medium and long-term outcome of phobic disorders because they are lost and disillusioned along the way. We must not forget them when evaluating the effectiveness of behaviour therapy in anxiety.

COGNITIVE THERAPY IN ANXIETY DISORDERS

Cognitive therapy was originally developed in the treatment of depression and involved the novel concept that the symptoms of this disorder might be a consequence of cognitive dysfunction rather than the cause of such dysfunction (Beck, 1976). Beck, who has the ability of Freud to formulate complex psychological ideas into simple straightforward language, suggested that much of depressive symptomatology could be classified in terms of cognitive errors such as irrational automatic intrusive thoughts (e.g. I am useless), inflexible primary assumptions concerning the individual oneself and/or his or her relationship with others (e.g. no-one has ever liked me) and cognitive distortions described under the catchy headings of selective abstraction, arbitrary inference, overgeneralisation, dichotomous thinking, and magnification or minimisation of thoughts. Together, Beck combined these in a cognitive triad consisting of three negatives, a negative view of oneself, one's interpretation of present feelings, and expectation of the future.

It quickly became apparent, as the reader who has taken on the general theme of this book will have predicted already, that the treatment could easily be transferred to the treatment of anxiety and phobias with relatively little modification (Beck et al., 1985). The main difference was that it was not the negative cognitive triad of depression that was being generated by cognitive dysfunction, but a threatening triad of catastrophisation, alarm and insecurity that constituted anxiety generation.

The consequences of this triad are demonstrated in Fig. 7.4, which illustrates a type of cognitive dysfunction often found in panic. The errors in thinking are obvious; it is wrong to take the evidence of your bodily feelings too literally and to assume you have a major physical disease, but all too often patients follow this path and "catastrophise" their disorder. The task of the cognitive therapist is to help the patient to

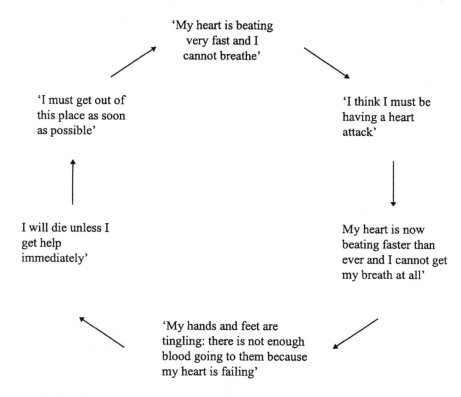

'My heart is beating
very fast and I
cannot breathe'

'I must get out of
this place as soon
as possible'

'I think I must be
having a heart
attack'

I will die unless I
get help
immediately'

My heart is now
beating faster than
ever and I cannot get
my breath at all'

'My hands and feet are
tingling: there is not enough
blood going to them because
my heart is failing'

Fig. 7.4 The positive feedback following misinterpretation of severe anxiety.

identify these errors, not by instruction but by collaboration, and then replace them with less dysfunctional thoughts (Clark, 1986).

The main principles of cognitive therapy, recently outlined by Brewin (1996), emphasise that different elements of the treatment are generalised or finely focused, and may modify both consciously accessible beliefs and unconscious ones represented in memory. There is also some evidence that cognitive procedures directed at changing misinterpretations of bodily sensations can reduce panic attack frequency as well as dysfunctional thoughts about disease, and unless these are addressed, there is no improvement (Salkovskis *et al.*, 1991).

Comparisons of cognitive therapy and behaviour therapy in generalised anxiety disorder have shown cognitive therapy to be generally superior with fewer drop-outs from treatment (Butler *et al.*, 1993; Power *et al.*, 1990). Cognitive therapy is also effective in irritable bowel syndrome (Greene and Blanchard, 1994; Payne and Blanchard, 1995), in social phobia (Heimberg and Barlow, 1991), in panic (Lidren *et al.*, 1994) and hypochondriasis (Warwick, 1989).

The place of cognitive therapy and exposure treatments has been well highlighted by a study which showed that exposure therapy is not effective in the treatment of panic disorder alone while cognitive therapy is not effective in agoraphobia alone (van den Hout *et al.*, 1994). Of course they can be combined and much of the effectiveness of the hybrid treatment, cognitive-behaviour therapy rests on its ability to correct dysfunctional thoughts and test out new methods of coping behaviour (Gelder, 1986).

INTERPERSONAL PSYCHOTHERAPY

This form of psychotherapy was developed as a research control treatment in conjunction with pharmacological research (Klerman, 1988) and has never been as popular as it should be. This is partly because almost all new psychological treatments are headed by a charismatic figure who is a strong proselytiser for the new approach (Freeman, personal communication) and interpersonal psychotherapy is more a treatment designed by a research group with few strong proponents.

In fact, the treatment is an efficient and well-organised summary of the essentials of psychotherapeutic treatment stripped of much of its less proven dynamic components. There has been little published work on interpersonal psychotherapy in anxiety, but in depression it has held its head up high when compared with other treatments. Thus, for example, in the National Institute of Mental Health Treatment of Depression Collaborative Research Program (discussed more fully below), in the subgroup of patients who were more severely depressed with greater functional impairment, there was greater evidence of the effectiveness of interpersonal psychotherapy compared with other psychological treatments (Elkin *et al.*, 1989). What was also interesting was that the key outcome measures said to be addressed by each of the therapies showed no evidence of selectivity; a good treatment was good in all respects, not just in the area of alleged expertise (Imber *et al.*, 1990).

BIOFEEDBACK

Biofeedback is an application of operant conditioning in which human subjects are given feedback on their autonomic nervous system functioning such as sweating or forehead muscle tension (such as, for example, converting the skin resistance or voltage of the electromyogram into an audible tone that increases in pitch with increasing intensity). With this extra information available, patients are better able to learn approaches that reduce the physiological changes and thereby reduce anxiety. Unfortunately, despite initial high hopes for such treatment, it has turned out to be a damp squib, with biofeedback of skin resistance changes having no real value and only the electromyogram showing some positive results (Rice and Blanchard, 1982). It is particularly helpful in the treatment of persistent headache (Blanchard *et al.*, 1990).

ANXIETY MANAGEMENT AND RELAXATION TRAINING

Anxiety management training is a formal procedure introduced by Suinn and Richardson (1971) and further developed in Oxford by Michael Gelder, which can be described as a form of combined relaxation and behavioural training. It was developed primarily as a treatment for generalised anxiety disorder and is undoubtedly effective in the condition (Butler *et al.*, 1987) but has no special advantages over cognitive and behavioural therapy with a high recurrence rate after treatment (Butler *et al.*, 1991, Butler, 1993).

Relaxation training, particularly progressive relaxation, first developed by Wolpe (1958), with some derivation from Jacobson's instructions to aid muscular relaxation (1939), involves up to six sessions of progressively greater relaxation training, and is a useful, if basic, treatment for anxiety which compares well with biofeedback (Canter *et al.*, 1975), and is better than control treatment or placebo tablets in panic disorder (Taylor *et al.*, 1982). A variant of this treatment, applied relaxation, which involves control of breathing and the induction of positive mental imagery, has been claimed to be superior to progressive relaxation and is possibly as effective as exposure and cognitive therapy (Ost *et al.*, 1993).

HYPNOTHERAPY

Hypnotherapy is one of the oldest treatments in psychiatry. It was developed by Mesmer, a Viennese physician, who developed dramatic cures in patients by talking to them in a commanding voice, inducing sleep in some cases, and laying his hands over the body to redistribute "magnetic fluid" within the body. He called this phenomenon "animal magnetism"; others called it Mesmerism (a word that has persisted in the language) and, when a special commission set up by Louis XVI of France (one of his last acts before the French revolution) reported that animal magnetism did not exist, poor old Mesmer was dumped and labelled a charlatan. In fact, the power of suggestion demonstrated by Mesmer has therapeutic value and had a period of respectability in the hands of Charcot in Paris and Freud in Vienna in the late nineteenth century. However, it has fallen from grace in the past 50 years. It has rarely been tested in controlled treatment trials and, when it has been, it performs less well than other psychological treatments (e.g. Marks *et al.*, 1966).

Despite this, it may have a place as an adjunctive therapy in anxiety disorders. Conditions which are prone to placebo effects are also helped by hypnosis, as both are influenced by suggestion. Some patients who prefer a passive authoritarian approach to treatment find it difficult to come to terms with the collaborative therapies such as cognitive-behaviour therapy. The fixed didactic approach of hypnosis, and the passive reception of treatment, are appealing and may be of particular value in getting the patient beyond the first stage of psychological therapy. Post-hypnotic suggestions may also be helpful in maintaining compliance.

EYE MOVEMENT DESENSITISATION

This is, at first sight, and also at second sight, a curious treatment for anxiety disorders. It involves the use of saccadic eye movements (scanning from side to side) and has been used almost entirely in the treatment of post-traumatic stress disorder. The procedure involves asking patients to focus their minds on an important feature of a traumatic experience (e.g. the scene after a major motor accident) while at the same time performing rhythmic saccadic eye movements. This treatment is alleged to lead to dramatic changes, including "a lasting reduction of anxiety, changes in the cognitive assessment of the memory, and cessation of flashbacks, intrusive thoughts, and sleep disturbances". Even more impressively, the treatment is said to be effective after only one session (Shapiro, 1989).

It is wise not to dismiss a treatment too readily when it appears to have no apparent physiological or psychological basis; most of the treatment in psychiatry is based on empiricism. Nevertheless, until evidence from rigorous treatment trials is available this must be regarded as an experimental procedure only.

SUBLIMINAL EXPOSURE TREATMENT

We only perceive (i.e. register consciously) a small proportion of the many sensations impinging on our nervous systems. Many of our feelings or actions that appear to be spontaneous are a consequence of the perception of stimuli, both external and internal, of which we are either unaware or which we appreciate at such a low level that we have to re-examine our experiences to detect them. Francis Galton, the father of fingerprinting and medical statistics, was amazed to find how much of his thinking was generated by apparently random thoughts and events and, by attending to this, discovered the phenomenon of free association. Anxious people, particularly those who are phobic, have the opposite problem; they are almost too sensitive to the stimuli that others ignore and this reinforces their anxiety.

The idea that exposure to anxious stimuli, the cornerstone of phobic treatment, might be aided by subliminal exposure to the same stimuli, is based on the same notion as desensitisation. There is also the apparent advantage of getting beyond the cognitive dysfunction that may perpetuate the anxiety, "the pale cast of thought" that may sabotage all attempts to resolve the anxious state. In practice the results have been encouraging but have not been followed through, so it is difficult to know if the therapy is of real value.

Subliminal messages have long been imbued with concern that they could be used to manipulate our minds to make us do things that we would otherwise deplore. The same was said about hypnosis in the past, but no-one exposed to either of these procedures acts in a way which is fundamentally different from normal. In fact, much of the claims about the impact of subliminal stimulation was overstated (e.g. putting the message "buy Blogg's ice cream" as every 32nd exposure in a cine-film does not increase the consumption of ice-cream at the interval), but there is no doubt that subliminal perception (the perception of a stimulus administered below the threshold of consciousness) is a genuine phenomenon (Dixon, 1971).

In personal experiments we have used cine-film at low levels of illumination and at high background levels of anxiety to induce or reduce anxiety. This was shown to be useful in agoraphobic patients who had not responded to other treatments (Tyrer et al., 1978) and both supraliminal and subliminal exposure were associated with improvement to a greater extent than a control film. Interestingly, the agoraphobic patients showed little provocation of anxiety under subliminal conditions (Lee and Tyrer, 1981) yet improved their avoidance of phobic situations. A later study showed that gradually increasing the illumination of the anxiety inducing films from subliminal to supraliminal levels (fading) was significantly more effective than supraliminal and control exposure in reducing phobic fear (Lee et al., 1983) and might be the best way of giving this treatment.

MEDITATION AND OTHER RELATED TREATMENTS

Meditation, a treatment made famous, or notorious, depending on your point of view, by the Maharishi Mahesh Yogi, is thought of mainly as a life-enhancement procedure. Like many other forms of psychological treatment akin to relaxation it is effective (Smith *et al.*, 1995) but it has not be tested adequately against the other standard treatments described in this chapter except in non-clinical populations. Other approaches, such as the Japanese treatment, shiatsu, and acupuncture, are likely to have good anti-anxiety effects but the necessary controlled trials to formalise this efficacy have not yet been carried out.

SELF-HELP

Self-help is a potentially ground-breaking treatment for anxiety disorders; the main problem is the best form of delivering it. When one considers the large number of people with anxiety disorders in the population at any one time (7–14% of the population), it is clear that there will never be sufficient therapists to treat it using psychological means, nor sufficient physicians to treat with pharmacological ones (even if this approach was considered desirable). Self-help has been shown in a number of studies to be helpful, with less demand for drug prescriptions (benzodiazepines) when administered in primary care (Donnan *et al.*, 1990) and though in general, it is not as good and effective as cognitive approaches (Payne and Blanchard, 1995), it has been shown in a personal study (Tyrer *et al.*, 1993) to be more effective in the medium term (10–52 weeks) than cognitive-behaviour therapy and antidepressant drug treatment, but only in patients with no personality disorder.

With newer forms of technology, it is now possible to develop self-help packages which are quite sophisticated and include all the elements of instructions involved in live therapy. In its simplest form, self-help is given as bibliotherapy, self-teaching reading material (e.g. Weekes, 1962), and this has been shown to be effective in treating panic (Lidren *et al.*, 1994). It is now conventional advice to suggest that initial therapy for anxiety, particularly generalised anxiety disorder, should include self-help (Lader *et al.*, 1992) but all too often it is not put into practice.

COMBINATION OF PSYCHOLOGICAL AND PHARMACOLOGICAL THERAPY

In general, the data support the combination of pharmacological and psychological treatments in anxiety. Thus the combination of buspirone and cognitive-behaviour therapy is more effective than either alone (Cottraux *et al.*, 1995); cognitive-behaviour therapy combined with diazepam is superior to either diazepam or cognitive behaviour therapy alone in the treatment of generalised anxiety disorder (Power *et al.*, 1990). In one recent large study involving meta-analysis (the combination of results from several trials) of controlled studies of the treatment of agoraphobia and panic conditions, the combination of antidepressants with exposure *in vivo* was the most effective treatment out of seven types of intervention (van Balkom *et al.*, 1997).

Psychological treatments may also help in pharmacological treatment problems. Cognitive-behaviour therapy has been shown to aid benzodiazepine withdrawal (Tyrer *et al.*, 1985; Otto *et al.*, 1993) and could be used more commonly in this condition. One of the reasons for this might be that patients who attribute their improvement, rightly or wrongly, to drug therapy, are the most likely to relapse after withdrawal (Basoglu *et al.*, 1994); cognitive-behaviour therapy may alter this perception.

RELAPSE AFTER PSYCHOLOGICAL TREATMENTS

Although the outcome of treatment with cognitive therapy is generally good, it may have been overstated in some quarters. Many patients have a return of symptoms and need further treatment after the main course has been completed, and those with comorbid disorders are more likely to have further problems (Brown and Barlow, 1992, 1995). In a recent review, Durham and Allan (1993) point out that psychological therapy generally results in modest improvement only, as only around 50% of patients achieve normal functioning with no tendency to relapse. Not surprisingly, if patients are recruited from primary care and are taking no medication, they tend to have a better outcome. The effects of cognitive therapy also tend to be long-lasting, but the treatment is generally less effective in those with co-occurring personality disorders compared with drug treatment (Tyrer *et al.*, 1993), although in the short-term little difference is shown (Dreessen *et al.*, 1994).

Despite these mixed findings, there is no doubt that relapse is much more frequent after drug therapy than psychological treatments, of which cognitive therapy has been the most studied. One of the major problems with drug treatment is that it is a passive exercise involving the patient little, except with regard to compliance with the drug regime. If the expectation develops that no progress can be made without external help, such as drugs, a condition called learned helplessness may develop and affect other behaviour (Seligman, 1975).

We have constantly pointed out the similarities between anxiety and depression in this book, and the problems of efficacy of different treatments and the likelihood of relapse are likely to be similar in both disorders. In the National Institute of Mental Health Treatment of Depression Collaborative Research Program, probably the most expensive treatment trial to date not mounted by a pharmaceutical company, in 250 patients with major depression (a condition which is more minor than major as the criteria required to diagnose it are very generous), the treatment phase consisted of 16 weeks of randomly assigned treatment with cognitive- behaviour therapy, interpersonal therapy, imipramine hydrochloride and clinical management (CM), or placebo plus CM. Follow-up assessments were conducted at 6, 12, and 18 months after treatment. Of the patients entering treatment and having follow-up data, those who recovered and remained well during follow-up (with no relapse of depression) did not differ significantly among the four treatments: these figures were 30% for cognitive behaviour therapy, 26% for interpersonal psychotherapy, 19% for those having imipramine plus CM, and 20% for those receiving placebo plus CM (Shea *et al.*, 1992). These figures suggest (but are not significant) that in the longer term, the psychotherapies are better than antidepressants; much of the comparison data suggesting better effects of drugs involves a much shorter time span.

Whilst it would be wrong to extrapolate from depression to anxiety disorders, there is abundant evidence that findings in one condition tend to be reflected in the other, with only minor modifications between them.

THE PLACE OF PSYCHOLOGICAL TREATMENTS IN THE TREATMENT OF ANXIETY

For the motivated patient, the brief cognitive therapies are at least as good as any other treatments for anxiety (Andrews, 1990; Clark, 1990) and it is likely that interpersonal psychotherapy is not far behind. The research data, taken together, look more impressive than is probably the case, as they refer to treatment given by enthusiastic therapists who are excellently trained, but these are not the norm in a clinical service. When other therapists, particularly those in the nursing profession who are likely to be the main protagonists of such treatment in the future, are involved in treatment the benefits are limited from interventions by untrained or less competent therapists (Kingdon *et al.*, 1996). However, when trained, psychiatrists, nurse practitioners and psychologists normally working with pharmacological treatments are effective in administering such treatments (Welkowitz *et al.*, 1991).

It is reasonable to conclude, with EM Forster on democracy, two cheers can be given for psychological treatments for anxiety but a much greater programme of education and self-help is needed to bring it up to three. When even a body such as Drugs and Therapeutics Bulletin (1993), which might be considered to have some tendency to choose drug treatment rather than others, was able to conclude in a recent review of the treatment of all anxiety disorders that "psychological treatments are an effective alternative to drug therapy for patients with acute reactions to stress, generalised anxiety disorder, agoraphobia and panic disorders, and in general result in a lower relapse rate once treatment is stopped", the message is being well advertised. This is a staggering achievement for a group of treatments that has very little financial muscle behind it. Many times in this account, I have referred to insufficient evidence being available to conclude whether psychological approaches are effective or not. This is true, but when the same problem faces a drug treatment, it is almost always in the interests of the pharmaceutical industry to fund the appropriate investigations to answer the question, and the sums of money may be very large indeed. The psychological treatments have no such advantages and it is a measure of their stature that they have been able to prove their worth with the help of a patchwork of support from charities, research councils and government funding. This support is fickle and unreliable, but it has one advantage summarised in the words of Ernest Rutherford, the father of atomic physics, "we have no money, so we will have to think".

Chapter 8

OUTCOME OF ANXIETY DISORDERS

A good diagnosis is like gold dust: it should be able to indicate the cause of a disorder, its natural history, its pathology, its symptomatology, and the correct intervention or treatment. It should also be able to predict outcome, both in terms of outcome in the absence of intervention (natural history) and also when an ideal treatment has been administered. The recent development of exciting new diagnoses in anxiety has led to interest that there may be important differences in their outcome and that of depression and other related disorders. Certainly there should be differences in at least some respects if the diagnoses are to be regarded as clinically useful. It is also important to know what to tell people with these disorders when they ask what will happen to them. Doctors have a tendency to resort to platitudes such as "it is impossible to tell because so much depends on how motivated you are to change" or delphic utterances such as "you will achieve a state of equilibrium that is right for you"; this is not appropriate when there are answers available.

The ideal course of anxiety disorders according to the present classification system is demonstrated in Fig. 8.1. The specific diagnoses of anxiety each have, if they are clinically useful, specific treatments and each of these is successful, if not at first, at least later. As none of these conditions is permanent, it is therefore to be expected that all would lead to sufficient improvement to be called recovery.

This is therefore the target for all treatments, but of course treatments are not always given at the right time and place and so the outcome of disorders is a mix of the consequences of intervention and the natural

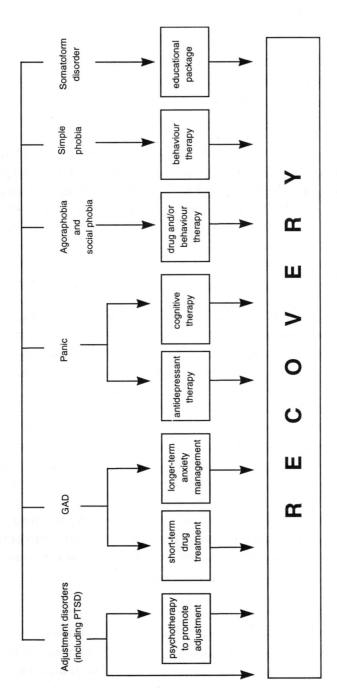

Fig. 8.1 The ideal course of anxiety disorders.

history of the condition. If there were important differences between the natural histories of the different anxiety and neurotic disorders, they should therefore be reflected in their outcomes, particularly if the outcome is a long-term one.

The best form of comparison is to take the disorders as they present, preferably a consecutive cohort, and to follow them up as completely as possible. In order to allow for the possibility that different treatments will alter outcome because they have different effects, it would also be appropriate to randomise treatment to each of the different diagnoses. However, this procedure, however well justified scientifically, would be regarded as intolerable by any self-respecting ethics committee as it would not allow the clinical freedom to give any treatment that might become necessary over the course of the follow-up period.

When one examines the literature on the outcome of anxiety disorders, there are very few studies that even go part of the way towards achieving these requirements. We have recently carried out a systematic review of the outcome of anxiety and depressive disorders (Emmanuel *et al.*, 1998) and, apart from the Nottingham Study of Neurotic Disorder referred to earlier, there have been no outcome comparisons of different anxiety disorders yet published. The primary intentions of the review were to investigate whether: (i) the outcome of specific anxiety disorders differed from each other; (ii) the outcome of anxiety disorders differed from those of depressive ones; and (iii) the outcome of single anxiety and depressive disorders differed from that of combined anxiety and depression (dual diagnosis). Although, originally, it was hoped to compare the outcome of the many diagnoses within the depressive and anxiety rubric, such studies were few and most comparisons were between depressive and anxiety disorders in general. The expectations of the investigators at the outset was that no important differences in outcome would be identified with the possible exception of a worse outcome in combined anxiety-depressive (dual) diagnoses.

DEFINITION OF OUTCOME

Before outcome can be measured satisfactorily, we need to be clear exactly what it is. A recent review of the outcome of depression (Puccinelli and Wilkinson, 1994) found it impossible to combine studies of outcome in a satisfactory way because the definitions of outcome were so different. Some studies record outcome as the presence or absence of illness (measured by whether they have a psychiatric diagnosis at follow-up), whereas others include measures of social functioning, current treatment received, and whether or not the subject is in gainful employment. There are also differences between studies which record outcome as the state the patient is in at the time of follow-up, irrespective of how they have been earlier, and those that record symptoms and other variables throughout the period of follow-up and thereby measure outcome longitudinally (e.g. Warshaw *et al.*, 1994). Here we shall assume that outcome refers usually to how the patient has been in the last six months, and that symptoms and social functioning are normally both included in the assessment of outcome.

It is also not entirely clear what period should elapse before outcome as a variable can be measured. The term is used in a vague sort of way to describe anything that is recorded some time after base-line measurements or an intervention has been made. However, good outcome studies are thought of normally in years rather than in weeks or months. Another important issue is drop-outs. It is quite possible for authors to present an outstanding set of data on a sample of patients seen at baseline (n) with the condition under test, but if there is steady attrition from this time onwards there may only be n/5 seen at follow-up. Most of these will have been treated and are probably compliant with what has been given (as after all, they are compliant enough to be available for research interview). They are, therefore, likely to be a specially selected group that is not representative of the condition as a whole; the value of such data, if drop-out rates are large, must therefore be very questionable.

STUDIES OF OUTCOME

In addition to comparative studies, there have been many individual follow-up studies of individual anxiety disorders. It is worthwhile discussing these separately, despite the difficulty in comparing across studies, because the populations included are so different.

OUTCOME OF PANIC DISORDER AND PHOBIAS

Studies in these disorders are difficult to separate because most research workers see patients with panic disorder when they already have well-developed phobias, mainly agoraphobia but also social phobias. This is particularly important if the additional (comorbid) condition contributes towards outcome, and, as we shall find, most certainly do. Roy-Byrne and Cowley (1995) have recently reviewed 16 studies and have encountered the many problems outlined above, of which the most difficult to overcome is the definitional one of outcome.

In our own work we have recorded outcome in terms of symptoms, functioning and health service usage, as these are all important elements that are to some extent independent. This leads to patients being allocated into one of four outcome groups (which apply after any duration of outcome):

- No appreciable symptoms or handicap created by psychiatric problems and no contact with either general practice or psychiatric services since initial period of care (usually lasting up to 9 months);
- A combination of some psychiatric symptoms of mild severity with some social dysfunction and occasional contact with health services for these problems but generally well;
- Persistent mild or occasional severe symptoms with greater social dysfunction and frequent contact with services for psychiatric problems for more than half of time of follow-up;
- Persistent symptoms after initial period of care, often severe and leading to severe social handicap, and usually associated with frequent contact with all forms of psychiatric service as well as with primary care and accident and emergency services (Seivewright et al., 1998).

This four-point scale will be used throughout this chapter and although relatively few studies have used all three measures of outcome, the reported findings at least have some measure of consistency.

Roy-Byrne and Cowley (1995) found that most studies showed improvement in panic symptoms to a greater extent than other symptoms. Around one in two of the patients in the studies had no panic attacks at the time of follow-up and this at first sight seems impressive.

However, in most studies panic attacks are recorded over a relatively short time period (often only for three weeks as in the original diagnosis of panic disorder in DSM-III) and the figures can be deceptive. In the Nottingham Study of Neurotic Disorder, for example, we found that 77% of patients with an original diagnosis of panic disorder had no panic attacks in the three weeks before assessment at 2 years, but there was an average of 1.7 attacks for each patient in the group and one patient experienced 35 attacks in the previous three weeks.

Phobic symptoms show much less improvement, with only one in three patients having no phobic symptoms at follow-up (Roy-Byrne and Cowley, 1995). Generalised anxiety also shows much less change with very few patients showing significant change in generalised anxiety despite having many fewer panic attacks (Nagy *et al.*, 1989). Depression, which is present at the same time as the panic disorder at base-line, has a negative effect on outcome in most studies and, not surprisingly, is associated with greater numbers of depressive episodes during the follow-up period. Around 30% of all patients with panic disorder develop major depression subsequently (Roy-Byrne and Cowley), and this number becomes much greater if longer follow-up periods are used, with Vollrath and Angst (1989) finding that 50% of patients developed depressive episodes after seven years of follow-up and even in those with "pure panic disorder" at outset, 42% developed depressive episodes. This is further evidence of the close links between depression and anxiety identified in genetic studies (Roy *et al.*, 1995). In those studies in which personality status has been measured at onset, the presence of personality disorder is highly predictive of a worse outcome (Noyes *et al.*, 1990; Faravelli and Albanesi, 1987).

Not surprisingly, those with more severe symptoms are more likely to have greater social dysfunction but this is not universal. Roy-Byrne and Cowley (1995) also examined the predictors of outcome and found that panic attack frequency has no value, and comorbidity with either agoraphobia, depression or personality disorder was predictive of a worse outcome, with personality disorder showing the strongest effects. As personality disorder is associated with persistent social dysfunction (Tyrer and Casey, 1993); this also brings social handicaps into the frame. Alcohol dependence may also be a secondary complication of panic disorder and then needs attention in its own right (Lepola, 1994).

We are therefore left with the conclusion that although patients with panic disorder often lose their panic symptoms, they continue to have other problems and their course is "characterised by fluctuating anxiety and depressive symptoms" (Albus and Schiebe, 1993). In the terms of our outcome scores, pure panic disorder has outcome 2, and if agoraphobia, depression or personality disorder are present this falls to outcome 3, with possibly outcome 4 if all comorbid conditions are present together.

Those with primarily phobic symptoms have a less satisfactory outcome than those with panic. Although those treated with behaviour therapy make significant gains, less than 20% can be described as recovered and many still need (or demand) further treatment for their symptoms (Emmelkamp and Kuipers, 1979; Lelliott *et al.*, 1987). The overall outcome for this group (and it is important to note that this is likely to be a selected sample as they are all involved in treatment) is between 2 and 3 on our outcome scale.

OUTCOME OF GENERALISED ANXIETY DISORDER

The outcome of generalised anxiety disorder is generally less good than other symptomatic variants such as depressive, phobic and panic disorders. As discussed earlier, this may be because it is linked closely to avoidant or anxious personality disorder and so, like all personality disorders, they tend to persist over time. Despite this, there have been few studies of the outcome of this condition, possibly because it is less glamorous than the other anxiety disorders that have consumed so much attention recently because of their novelty and aspirations to clinical insight.

One problem is that so few groups with a specific diagnosis of generalised anxiety disorder have been followed up for an adequate length of time. However, some earlier studies have examined conditions under the general rubric of anxiety that can clearly be linked to generalised aspects of the condition. Thus Kerr *et al.* (1972) found that "tension", one of the cardinal features of generalised anxiety disorder, was the strongest negative predictor of outcome after nearly 4 years, and Ormel *et al.* (1993), using a sample identified from the Present State Examination (Wing *et al.*, 1974) in primary care patients (which include a preponderance of patients with generalised anxiety disorder) found that only 33% of those with anxiety had recovered (outcome 1) after 3.5 years (compared with 47% of those with an initial diagnosis of depression). An even lower figure of 12% recovery after 15–20 years was identified by Quinton *et al.* (1995) in a sample seen as children and also diagnosed using the Present State Examination. In a more recent study involving patients diagnosed formally as having generalised anxiety disorder, of 110 patients offered treatment and randomly allocated, 66 were followed up and of these, only three (5%) were judged to have recovered (outcome 1) and 20 (30%) were considerably improved (outcome 2) (Durham *et al.*, 1994).

Generalised anxiety disorder appears therefore to be a persistent condition that is even present to some degree many years after initial diagnosis. The diagnostic problem of generalised anxiety disorder being a heterogeneous "dustbin" diagnosis (Hoehn-Saric, 1982; Hoehn-Saric and McLeod, 1985) makes further interpretation difficult.

OUTCOME OF ANXIOUS PERSONALITIES

The difficulty is separating anxiety as a personality trait from anxiety as a symptom of disorder, has been mentioned many times earlier in this book and so it is appropriate to look at the outcome of those who have anxious personalities (avoidant personality in DSM-IV). There is relatively little work on this subject as the outcome of these disorders is difficult to evaluate in view of the recency of diagnostic identification of this group. However, in what could be called proxy evidence, studies of the prevalence of personality disorder in different age groups can be used to predict what the outcome is liable to be when examined prospectively. In populations of randomly selected subjects and those attending psychiatric services, there is no evidence that anxious personalities are less common in older subjects and in this respect anxiety differs from all other personality disorders, which tend to become less prevalent over time (Tyrer and Seivewright, 1988). Although there are claims that such personality disorder can be positively influenced by treatment, particularly with antidepressive drugs such as fluoxetine (Deltito and Stam, 1989) this needs much more investigation and a longer period of follow-up than has been carried out to date.

SYSTEMATIC REVIEW OF THE OUTCOME OF ANXIETY AND DEPRESSIVE DISORDERS

This review (Emmanuel *et al.*, 1998) was carried out using the recommended procedures for systematic reviews (stimulated largely by the work of the Cochrane collaboration, an international group set up in 1992 following the pioneering work of Archie Cochrane (an epidemiologist who died in 1987 after a lifetime of work devoted to developing better systems of determining the efficacy of health care)). A systematic review uses standardised procedures that allow the results of studies to be combined using the technique of meta-analysis so that informed conclusions can be made with the minimum of bias. To illustrate how this is done the procedure is described in some detail.

STAGE ONE - SEARCH

We searched all literature published in English in the MEDLINE® database from 1966–1997, using the terms anxiety disorders, depression and outcome, and, as a separate subject, randomised controlled trials. The search strategy was set in general terms to include all diagnoses of anxiety and depression so that all possible studies could be accessed. Two people examined the abstracts, titles and descriptor terms of all the papers identified in the electronic searches and those that were unsuitable (i.e. did not address the subject of the review adequately were discarded (if both people agreed), leaving a pool of potentially eligible studies.

STAGE TWO - IDENTIFICATION OF APPROPRIATE STUDIES

The procedure above identified a total of 44 possible original articles and, as an additional check, examination of all the references in these articles was carried out to see if any others had been missed from the original procedure, but no additional papers were found. The same authors independently evaluated these 44 articles and extracted the data from those considered to be appropriate for inclusion. Although the papers included in this review examined the "naturalistic outcome" of the diagnosis, in which some intervention has usually been given, the ideal studies for comparison of outcome are randomised and quasi-randomised controlled ones in which treatment is controlled (i.e. allowed for by randomisation), and so it was hoped that some of these would be identified too. (Otherwise the outcome could be the same for all the treatment groups if the appropriate "ideal treatment" had been given (Fig. 8.1)). Studies which only described the outcome of a single diagnosis, with no comparative element (discussed elsewhere in this Chapter) were excluded, as were studies addressing the outcome of any anxiety or depressive disorders in which comparison was only made with similar comorbid groups (e.g. anxiety vs anxiety plus personality disorder).

Thirty-six of the 44 articles were excluded for the following reasons:

(a) they were concerned with comorbidity only (14 papers), (e.g. Brown *et al.*, 1995, Lesser *et al.*, 1988)
(b) they did not include a comparison group with a separate diagnosis (nine papers) (e.g. Brown and Schulberg 1995; Noyes *et al.*, 1980)
(c) unclear diagnostic information at baseline (six papers) (e.g. Delini-Stula *et al.*, 1995)
(d) they were essentially review articles (four papers) (e.g. Roth and Argyle, 1988)
(e) they examined prognostic factors in outcome only
(f) the period of study was only five weeks (Johnstone *et al.*, 1980).

Of the eight studies, only one involved prospective randomisation of treatment across diagnostic groups — the Nottingham Study of Neurotic Disorder (Tyrer *et al.*, 1993) — and the specific outcome in this study is discussed later. Most of the studies gave no information about treatment during follow-up. Van Valkenberg *et al.* (1984) described an open "standard" treatment regime (antidepressants, benzodiazepines and various psychotherapeutic interventions) given across groups, but none of the other studies reported specific treatment schedules.

RESULTS

Meta-analysis is most easily carried out for dichotomous (yes/no) variables and the results for two of these, i.e. improvement to having no psychiatric diagnosis at the time of the outcome assessment, and its extreme converse outcome, no improvement between base-line and outcome assessments, are shown in Fig. 8.2, which includes a summary for (a) comparisons of anxiety vs depressive diagnoses, and (b) anxiety vs mixed anxiety/depression and depression vs mixed anxiety-depression.

The results showed clear evidence that comorbid anxiety-depressive diagnoses had a worse outcome than single anxiety and depressive ones and, to a somewhat lesser degree, that anxiety diagnoses had a worse outcome than depressive ones. These are demonstrated in Fig. 8.2 in which the combined results from the different studies are shown by the flattened diamond. When part of the diamond crosses the vertical line, this indicates absence of significance between the two comparative diagnoses; when the diamond is separated from the line, the two conditions have significantly different outcomes.

There is little doubt that the possession of a mixed anxiety-depressive diagnosis confers a worse outcome. It is important to emphasise in this context that a mixed diagnosis is different from the diagnosis of mixed anxiety-depression in ICD-10, as this is only allowed for "sub-syndromal" diagnoses (i.e. those that do not reach the criteria for either a depressive or an anxious diagnosis). The comorbid anxious-depressive group in Fig. 8.2 reaches the criteria for both anxiety and depressive diagnoses, and the clear position of the means to the left of the line indicates a worse outcome in the mixed group.

Despite the overall findings, there were some important differences between the individual studies. For example, one study that showed a worse outcome in patients with depressive disorder was that by

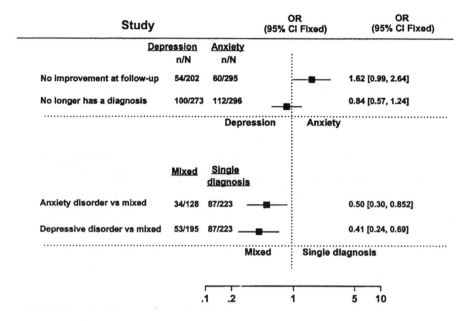

Fig. 8.2 Summary of results of systematic review of outcome of anxiety disorders compared with depressive ones (derived from Emmanuel *et al.*, 1998, with permission of the authors and the *British Journal of Psychiatry*). NB. The results of all studies qualifying for inclusion in the review are shown on the left. The graphical representation in the centre of the figure shows the odds ratio (OR) for the comparison anxiety vs depression (top two comparisons) or anxiety single, depression single vs mixed anxiety/depression (bottom two comparisons). The right-hand side of the figure shows the odds ratio and the confidence intervals (CI) (95%), which are also represented as the lines on either side of the means in the graphical representation. The vertical line in the graph shows the significance level of the findings. Those findings which have a mean score and confidence intervals which do not cross the line demonstrate significant differences; thus, in these comparisons anxiety patients are less likely than depressed ones to have no diagnosis at follow-up, and patients with single diagnoses have a much better outcome than mixed ones.

Murphy *et al.* (1986), which showed a worse outcome in depressive disorders. However, this finding may be explained by the different way of recording outcome in this study compared with the other ones. The recording method used regards discrete episodes of illness and continuous symptoms as equivalent and may therefore discriminate in favour of anxiety against depressive disorder, if, as other studies have shown, the depression is episodic.

ADDRESSING COURSE OF ILLNESS IN DETERMINATION OF OUTCOME

It is reasonable to argue that a single outcome measured at the endpoint of a study is a poor indicator of illness in general and disease burden in particular over the period of follow-up. One approach is to prospectively make frequent assessments of the patients during the study as discussed below (Tyrer *et al.*, 1993). Alternatively, it is possible to assess progress retrospectively (Schapira *et al.*, 1972, Murphy *et al.*, 1986) using a variety of methods. These can include assessments of social functioning, symptom severity and use of medication and can be combined in a weighted scoring system. Overall, these methods showed a similar outcome to the more straightforward categorical scoring of improvement and persistence of symptoms, although Schapira *et al.* (1972) reported that their scoring system reflected the fluctuations of the illness during the study period. Ormel *et al.* (1993) have described a multicategorical outcome measure to include patients with "borderline diagnoses", reporting that such a tool identified sub-clinical forms of both anxiety and depression, and Surtees and Barkley (1994) have usefully combined both current and past data in developing a Depression Outcome Scale (DOS) for long-term follow-up studies.

OUTCOME IN THE NOTTINGHAM STUDY OF NEUROTIC DISORDER

This study has been described earlier and differs from the others in this review because treatments were randomised at the beginning of the study and, despite the option of continuing with other treatments, was largely in the same mode (i.e. drug treatment, psychological treatment, or self-help) after two years (Tyrer *et al.*, 1993). The study also included a comparison of two anxiety diagnoses, generalised anxiety disorder and panic disorder, which was true for none of the other studies. Assessors were also blind to the initial diagnosis of each patient when they made their assessments. The results showed some differences between the diagnoses at different points in the study, but they were largely explained by factors that might be independent of the diagnostic process. Dysthymic disorder showed less improvement than panic disorder and generalised anxiety disorder with regard to anxiety symptoms in the first ten weeks of the study (Tyrer *et al.*, 1988b) but this difference was not shown subsequently. Over the course of the next two years, the patients with dysthymic disorder fared somewhat worse than those with the other two diagnoses but not significantly so (Fig. 8.3) and the outcome scores at two and five years showed no important differences between diagnostic groups (Table 8.1) (Seivewright *et al.*, 1998).

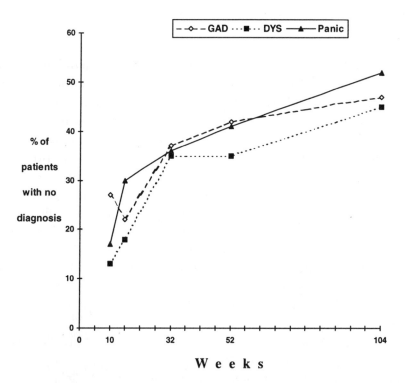

Fig. 8.3 Percentage of patients with an initial diagnosis of generalised anxiety disorder (GAD) (n = 59), dysthymic disorder (n = 56), and panic disorder (n = 66) receiving no diagnosis at different times of follow-up.

Table 8.1 Outcome of Patients with Generalised Anxiety Disorder (GAD) and Panic Disorder after Two and Five Years

Initial diagnosis		Percentage recovered		Percentage with additional diagnosis at two years		
	n	2 years	5 years	major depression	agoraphobia*	dysthymia**
GAD	53–58	47	60	9	6	11
Panic	62–63	52	56	11	18	2

* χ^2 = 2 85 (after Yates correction), P = 0.09
** χ^2 = 3.2 (after Yates correction), P = 0.07

The patients with generalised anxiety disorder are more likely to develop dysthymia and those with panic more likely to become agoraphobic (although this does not quite reach significance) but overall outcome is similar.

The slightly worse outcome of the depressive group in the Nottingham Study of Neurotic Disorder reduced the overall finding that depressive disorders in general had a better outcome than anxiety ones. However, it is important to realise that dysthymic disorder is not typical of depressive disorders as a whole (Akiskal, 1983; World Psychiatric Association, 1995). The diagnosis requires depressive symptoms to have been present for most of the past two years and so naturally will tend to include patients with a poorer outcome, at least in the shorter term. The patients with dysthymic disorder also had a higher proportion with personality disorder (51%) compared with panic disorder (31%) and generalised anxiety disorder (29%) (Tyrer et al., 1990b), and as personality disorder in general is associated with a worse outcome (Greer and Cawley, 1966; Perry et al., 1987; Shea et al., 1990; Brown and Barlow, 1992), it might be predicted that dysthymic patients would not improve as much as others.

However, taking the results as a whole both questions asked in this review had clear answers. Anxiety disorders have a worse outcome than depressive ones, and dual diagnosis of anxiety and depression has a worse outcome than either anxiety or depression alone. Most of the eight studies included patients with a dual anxiety and depressive diagnosis, which suggests that the way in which we carry out diagnosis in these disorders is generally inefficient and a better way of identifying those with worse outcome is urgently needed. Nevertheless, the finding that the long-term outcome is predicted successfully by initial diagnosis indicates that, whatever the confusion created by the high degree of overlap between anxiety and depression in follow-up studies (e.g. Kendell, 1974), the initial diagnosis of anxiety or depression is useful.

However, as already noted, the criteria for measuring outcome remain unsatisfactory and, in the absence of consensus or a theoretically driven definition, are likely to remain confused and arbitrary (Puccinelli and Wilkinson, 1994). If the outcome of anxiety disorders was a persistent but mild continuation of symptoms, and the outcome of depression an episodic but with more serious handicap during illness, the measurement of outcome at a fixed point in time, without taking into account the course of illness, might unfairly favour the depressive group.

Some evidence (e.g. Schapira et al., 1972) that anxiety disorders are more likely to be made in the presence of personality disorder may influence differences in outcome. However, as already noted, the Nottingham Study of Neurotic Disorder involved patients with dysthymia with high rates of personality disorder and it is interesting in this study that the results were in the opposite direction. The generally worse outcome in neurotic and depressive disorder in patients with personality disorder is now well-established (Shea et al., 1990; Reich and Vasile, 1993, Quinton et al., 1995) and so premorbid personality status may need to be taken into account in future enquiries.

The finding that patients with a dual diagnosis have a worse outcome than those with a diagnosis of anxiety alone, who in turn have a worse outcome than those with depression alone, suggests that attempts to give separate diagnostic status to the combined group, such as the general neurotic syndrome (Tyrer, 1985; Andrews et al., 1990; Tyrer et al., 1992) have some merit. This is particularly relevant in the significant number of patients who "crossed over" diagnosis from anxiety to depression or vice-versa if they relapsed during follow up.

IATROGENIC PROBLEMS INFLUENCING OUTCOME

Iatrogenic disease is a disorder created by the intervention of a physician (or other therapist) and is doubly unfortunate if it persists to alter the outcome of a condition. The main therapies used in the treatment of anxiety, discussed fully in the previous two chapters, all have one major problem, the tendency to create dependence. Sometimes this dependence may be relatively mild, such as when an agoraphobic patient becomes reliant on a behaviour therapist and cannot continue progress when, for example, the therapist is on holiday. In psychotherapy, the finding that a patient only remains passably well when continuing treatment, and whenever it is withdrawn relapse occurs (transference cure) is another example. Anxious patients tend to be dependent and this complication of treatment is hardly unexpected.

However, when the treatment becomes extremely widespread, such as the use of benzodiazepines for anxiety treatment in the 1960s and 1970s in the UK, or currently in France and the United States, the problems created by dependence can become much greater. Follow-up studies are relatively few in number and difficult to interpret as they deal with a heterogeneous group of patients. In personal studies of patients who had putative dependence on benzodiazepines before withdrawal, the overall outcome was fairly good, with 21% having recovered (outcome 1) and 48% having improved moderately or to some extent (outcomes 2 and 3) (Holton and Tyrer, 1990, Holton et al., 1992), but older patients and those with personality disorder did less well (Holton et al., 1992). Ashton (1984, 1987) has also published follow-up data on her patients dependent on benzodiazepines but although these look more promising (70% coming within outcomes 1 and 2), she assessed outcome primarily in terms of benzodiazepine use and did not assess other areas of function. Patients taking benzodiazepines seem to have a continued need to take therapy of some sort and, in our own study, the fact that 76% took further benzodiazepines in the follow-up period (even if only for short periods) (Holton and Tyrer, 1990) suggests that once someone has been taking benzodiazepines long-term, it is very difficult for them to break the habit entirely, even if it is only for short-term use at times of stress. In this respect, however, alcohol may be different from the benzodiazepines as the ability of patients to restart and stop benzodiazepines almost at will suggests a lower dependence risk than alcohol.

SUMMARY

The conclusion of this review of outcomes of anxiety disorder is one of guarded optimism. The results of the systematic review are unlikely to be the consequence of an error or a source of systematic bias; the procedure adopted in this review was a standard one in evidence-based medicine (Sackett et al., 1996) and shows the value of diagnosis as a categorical decision. Despite some criticism of the diagnostic process made elsewhere in this book, the ability to make a clear-cut diagnosis of either an anxiety or depressive diagnosis and its comorbid equivalent, is an important one that generates important questions and answers that are inherent to good practice (Geddes and Harrison, 1997).

A person who presents with any anxiety disorder alone, with no other complicating features, is likely to have a good long-term outcome although he or she may not lose symptoms entirely. However, because the symptoms would be relatively mild in nature it is usually possible to make an adequate adjustment to them and for them to cause relatively little suffering.

The comparison with depression may lead to the conclusion that it better to have a depressive disorder than an anxiety one. This depends on one's point of view. The depressed patient may have less time ill, but when unwell, will be much more handicapped than the anxious person (Fig. 8.4). Whereas the anxious person will normally have learned mechanisms of coping with symptoms that can be put into operation without any difficulty, the person who has a relapse of depression is often overwhelmed by the symptoms to the extent of being "taken over" by them and therefore suffers much more. When the suffering can lead to self-harm and possible suicide it easy to conclude that, if given the choice, it is better to have an anxiety than a depressive disorder.

It is worth noting, of course, that not only diagnosis is important in determining outcome. Social factors, in the broadest sense, have a major

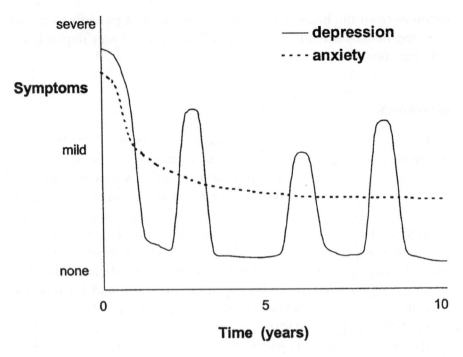

Fig. 8.4 General course of anxiety and depressive disorders illustrating variabilty in outcome.

influence on the outcome of anxiety and depressive disorders and are generally better predictors than formal diagnosis (Huxley *et al.*, 1979; Goldberg *et al.*, 1990; Brown *et al.*, 1992). (It is interesting that these authorities have tended to examine social factors in the absence of any assessment of personality status; the possibility of these findings being a consequence of personality disorder should also be considered.)

For those who have comorbidity with depression, personality disorder or obsessive compulsive disorder, the outcome is much less promising. This also appears to be the case if symptoms are likely to persist, remissions will be fewer and only a small minority will lose their symptoms entirely. There is a higher rate of deliberate self-harm (Vollrath and Angst, 1989) and it is likely that actual suicide rates will also be higher, as around 10% of those who harm themselves will commit suicide eventually (Nordentoft *et al.*, 1993). There is a particularly poor outcome in those who have a personality disorder within the anxious/fearful group (the general neurotic syndrome) in which the anxiety symptoms appear to be so intricately entwined with the personality that it is difficult to perceive of them as a separate disorder. The less satisfactory outcome for comorbid subjects with anxiety and depression also has implications for the diagnosis of mixed anxiety-depressive disorder. Wittchen and Essau (1993) recently examined data from a follow-up study in Munich and found a general prevalence of 1% for the sub-syndromal mixed anxiety-depressive disorder (although this figure can only be a guess since there are no clear criteria for diagnosing this disorder). Their additional findings that the disorder might be frequent in primary care settings, that the condition was often associated with substantial social handicaps, and that it was associated with high rates of health service input, are disturbing. Hecht *et al.* (1989, 1990) have also examined this phenomenon closely and concluded that the greater social handicaps in comorbidity are not entirely explained by greater symptoms or coincidental personality disturbance. These findings hint that mixed anxiety-depressive disorder might be at least as serious as single anxiety and depressive disorders and, since the general findings of this chapter indicate the prognosis for comorbid states is gloomy, their continued wait in the visitors' car park of the classification compound should soon be ended. Indeed, the gate may be about to open and the DSM classification could shortly admit a new member (Zinbarg *et al.*, 1994).

This has great implications for treatment. As discussed in Chapter six, it is difficult to be certain when people no longer need the treatment which originally may be effective for their condition. The only way in which we can test this at present is by the unsatisfactory technique of trial and error, gradually reducing the treatment and seeing whether the person relapses. For those with a single anxiety disorder this process should be carried out early, and for those with the comorbid disorders, it should be carried out late or, in some cases, not even tried at all. In making decisions, it is very important that the sufferer is brought into the discussion. Some people are perfectly happy taking medication for a life time for any type of disorder; others regard it with anathema. Increasingly, it is becoming clear that the right thing for the therapist to do is to put the prognostic cards on the table and work out a joint decision about length of treatment which can be reviewed at regular intervals (not least because the longer the period of review, the more information is available to make the final decision a more informed one).

Unfortunately, apart from one study in which panic and generalised anxiety disorder (Tyrer *et al.*, 1992) were compared, there were no comparisons of different anxiety disorders identified in this review. This is an important omission. We do not know which elements of anxiety are important in accounting for poor outcome — the development of agoraphobia, the influence of panic, the persistence of generalised anxiety, the complications of social phobia — and until comparative outcome studies are performed we can only speculate which of these are relevant. This is a pity, for if the new diagnostic groups within anxiety are to have lasting value, they need to be tested for their long-term predictive value as much as their short-term success in the selection of treatment strategies.

Chapter 9

RELATIONSHIP BETWEEN ANXIETY AND OTHER PSYCHIATRIC DISORDERS

Anxiety is an easy symptom to recognise but not necessarily useful in understanding the nature of a disorder. When our new medical students observe a patient presenting for the first time, either in a clinic or on a home visit, the question I put to them afterwards, "Would you like to summarise what you think might be wrong (with the patient)?" is all too frequently answered "He/she was anxious, restless or nervous", followed by a description of the objective signs of anxiety at interview. This is occasionally a correct summary, but much more often the patient has another disorder in which anxiety is only the external manifestation. The range of disorders is great and is illustrated in Fig. 9.1, in which the degree of overlap in the Venn diagram indicates the closeness of the association.

The reasons why anxiety can be so important in each of these disorders as a primary symptom are shown in Table 9.1. The nature of this relationship between anxiety and other disorders is a vexed question which taxes the minds of research workers and, as the rest of this chapter will show, makes us look foolish as the solutions we have proposed are more difficult to understand than the problem.

The conventional term now used for the association of one mental disorder with another is "comorbidity". This is not a satisfactory term for association, since comorbidity describes the presence of two independent and separate diseases in the same person at the same time (Feinstein, 1970). This is only one of many forms of association; there

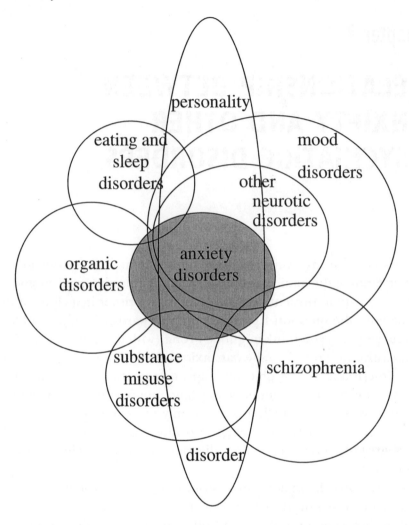

Fig. 9.1 Associations between anxiety and other psychiatric disorders.

are many others that indicate some causal connection between the different conditions, and some of these may be very complex (Lyons *et al.*, 1997). The most intimate form of association is one in which apparently different conditions are intrinsic components of the same disease or disorder, a form of association that could be classed as consanguinity (Tyrer, 1996).

Table 9.1 Mental Disorders that Can Present with Anxiety as the Main Symptom

ICD-10 group (WHO, 1992)	Disorder	Main presentation of anxiety
F0 (organic disorder)	Dementia	Early in course of disease when sufferer has awareness of loss of cognitive function but is trying to hide it
	Delirium	Anxiety associated with acute confusion in which a wide range of stimuli are perceived as potentially threatening
	Organic anxiety disorder	Acute episodes of anxiety (including panic) due to organic disease (e.g. epilepsy affecting temporal lobe)
F1 (substance use disorder)	Alcohol and drug dependence	Anxiety is a prominent component of the withdrawal syndrome characteristic of dependence and is often very severe (e.g. terror in delirium tremens)
F2 (schizophrenia and related disorders)	Early stages of schizophrenia or delusional disorder	"Delusional mood"; the anxiety associated with the notion that something odd is going on but the person does not know what it is
		Anxiety associated with paranoia (the anxiety of suspicion)
F3 (mood disorders)	All depressive disorders	Anxiety is almost invariably associated with depression to some degree
		In mixed anxiety-depression disorder it is given "subsyndromal status" (see text)
F4 (neurotic and stress disorders)	Obsessive-compulsive disorder	Anxiety is present at some stage in all these conditions
	Dissociative disorder	
	Somatisation disorder	
F5 (behavioural disorder with physiological disturbance)	Sleep disorder	Anxiety persistently associated with insomnia and with concern over weight
	Eating disorder	
F6 Personality disorder	Anxious personality disorder	Personality is a chronically anxious one

Table 9.2 Patterns of Association Between Playing Cards and Diseases

Relationship between cards	Description	Disease equivalent
None whatsoever	Random association	Comorbidity
Residue of previous relationships not removed by apparently random distribution	Pseudorandom association	Distant common vulnerability factors
Fixed pattern determined by previous manipulation of pack	False association	False comorbidity
Cards sorted in suits in ascending order	True association (secondary)	Primary and secondary disorder
Cards identical in notation	True association (common identity)	Consanguinity

The study of comorbidity in psychiatry is one of the fastest growing areas of the subject and it is important to establish the correct terminology at the outset before describing the specific diagnostic associations of anxiety. Imagine that you have come across a pack of playing cards for the first time and are observing players engaged in different games with them. Different forms of association will be observed at different times and these can be classified fairly easily (Table 9.2).

RANDOM ASSOCIATION (EQUIVALENT TO TRUE COMORBIDITY)

This pattern is observed most commonly when a pack of cards is shuffled and dealt to a number of players. The cards are distributed randomly and the cards in each hand, when dealt consecutively, do not have any intrinsic association. So whether the two of clubs appears next to the seven of diamonds or the queen of hearts is of no special significance. Just occasionally, the two of clubs may be placed next to a card which seems to be related in some way, such as the ace of clubs or the two of diamonds, but examination of the frequency with which this occurs shows that it does not take place more often than by chance.

PSEUDORANDOM ASSOCIATION

This pattern is demonstrated when the distribution of cards is apparently a random one but the pack has not been shuffled adequately and has the residue of previous associations present within the pack. This is sometimes found after many games of whist or bridge have been played with the same pack of cards. The players have repeatedly placed their cards into suits when playing each game and the shuffling procedure is not sufficient to remove this association entirely.

FALSE ASSOCIATION

This pattern is demonstrated when the pack of cards has been "doctored" to produce an apparently randomly distributed hand which is, in fact, artificially contrived for a particular purpose (e.g. to produce a winning hand at poker). Here there is no doubt that the association is a false one, but it appears to be random to the inexperienced or untrained.

TRUE ASSOCIATION (SECONDARY)

This association is found after a pack of cards has been distributed but has then been sorted by the player into standard groups for the purpose of playing the game. Thus in a game of bridge and whist the cards will be collected together in each of the four suits, spades, hearts, diamonds and clubs, with the cards in each suit placed in ascending or descending order. The observer will note immediately that this association is so unlikely to be a random one that it must have been created by some form of intervention. Of course there is sometimes a very rare event in which the cards are distributed in exactly the same pattern, entirely by chance, but the odds against this are very small. This type of association can be described as secondary as the cards have passed through an intermediate phase, reorganisation by the player, so that the game can be played more effectively.

TRUE ASSOCIATION (CONSANGUINITY)

The closest association is one of 100% concordance, or cards of identical function in this context. This is only noted normally when the two jokers are being used in the pack; the observer will notice they are identical in all essential respects. Although they may differ slightly in design, the important joker notation is the same and each card carries out the same function. However, in many card games the exact notation of some of the cards may be unimportant (e.g. vingt et un (Pontoon), where cards of the same spot value are regarded as equal for the purposes of the game. In these games, these cards could be regarded as being identical for the purposes of the game, even though they differ in appearance and numerical value.

FORMS OF ASSOCIATION BETWEEN ANXIETY AND OTHER PSYCHIATRIC DISORDERS

Random Association

The five forms of association found with the playing cards are replicated in the comorbidity of psychiatric disorders (Fig. 9.1) and is of particular relevance in the case of anxiety. True independent comorbidity is found when the frequency of association is no greater than would be expected by chance. Thus, if an epidemiological study found that anxiety disorders, which affect about 12–14% of the population at any one time (Regier *et al.*, 1990b, 1998; Meltzer *et al.*, 1994), and alcohol dependence, which affects around 10% (Kessler *et al.*, 1994), were found together in 1% of the population, the results could be presented as a chance association. Both are common disorders and therefore are likely to occur together.

As the reader might expect, studies showing such independence of diagnostic association are extremely rare and are notable for their splendid isolation in the psychiatric literature. The opposite is the case. In one recent study, National Comorbidity Survey in the United States, more than half of all lifetime psychiatric disorders in the population occurred in the 14% of the sample who had a history of three or more comorbid disorders (Kessler *et al.*, 1994). This degree of association in clinical populations is common and is sometimes explained by what is known as Berkson's bias, the increased tendency of persons with multiple diagnoses to seek and receive treatment and thus fall into study populations drawn from treatment sources. However, these findings are similar in epidemiological surveys, and in the National Morbidity study, less than 40% of those with a lifetime disorder had ever received professional treatment, and less than 20% of those with a recent disorder had been in treatment during the past 12 months. This is not the figure one would expect from Berkson's bias. The findings in all forms of study suggest that true comorbidity is so rare it can almost be dismissed as a clinical, as opposed to an epidemiological, phenomenon.

Pseudorandom Association

This type of association, whereby disorders appear to cluster together without any apparent inter-connection, but which on closer evaluation appear to be dependent on each other, is more common than often realised. Thus, if a person's early experiences lead to vulnerability to a range of psychiatric disorders when exposed to a specific stress in adult life, the consequences of such exposure could lead first to one of the stress and adjustment disorders, then to one or more of the major disorders that are subject to this vulnerability. When the vulnerability is regarded as a consequence of another condition, such as a personality disorder, yet another condition is added to the comorbidity grid. Brown and his colleagues (Brown *et al.*, 1992, 1993) have shown that much of the comorbidity of anxiety and depression in adult life could be (but not necessarily is) explained by such early vulnerabilities, often following exposure to major life stresses.

These distant causes can account for multiple comorbidity, but more recent ones can account for comorbidity with a single disorder, of which the anxiety disorders are amongst the most prominent. When one considers that anxiety is an emotion linked to uncertainty, and that uncertainty about one's own mental and physical health is more threatening than all others, it is entirely to be expected that anxiety disorders will be manifest at some time during the course of many psychiatric and physical conditions which are apparently independent of anxiety. The association of many disorders simultaneously or consecutively is a much reported observation best summarised in Shakespeare's words, "when sorrows come, they come not single spies, but in battalions".

False Association

This type of association can occur when the diagnostic descriptions of two disorders are faulty and conditions which should be quite separate are apparently linked together. The best example with the anxiety disorders is the association of social phobia and avoidant personality disorder. These conditions should really be quite separate, one being focused on symptoms of distress in social situations accompanied by avoidance of those situations in a specific and predictable manner; the other focusing on personality features of long-standing, in which there is general anxiety and fearfulness of the environment in general, so that lifestyle is restricted and attempts made to carve out a niche of settled security. These disorders have separate face validity, and every clinician can identify individuals who satisfy the characteristics of each disorder separately. However, after following the guidelines for diagnosis, the apparent comorbidity of these conditions is so high (around 75%) that it is more likely that they constitute the same rather than different disorders (Herbert *et al.*, 1992; Noyes *et al.*, 1995). It is also not surprising that avoidant personality disorder responds to the same treatment as does social phobia (Deltito and Stam, 1989), and that social phobia is a disease that apparently begins in early adolescence and persists throughout much of adult life (Merikangas and Angst, 1995; Mannuzza *et al.*, 1995) (i.e. has the typical time course of personality disorder).

Of course it is possible to argue that these two conditions are genuinely the same (i.e. constitute consanguinity as described below) and the decision whether the error in diagnosis is fundamental (the guidelines for diagnosis are wrong), or secondary (the two diagnoses have different descriptions but co-occur together to a much greater extent than expected) is often difficult to make at first. Further work may elucidate reasons for the association, and in the case of social phobia the separation of generalised social phobia (similar to avoidant personality disorder) and "non-generalised social phobia" (specific social phobia) may have some value (Mannuzza *et al.*, 1995). Other conditions which may illustrate false association with anxiety disorders include obsessive-compulsive disorder (Mellman and Uhde, 1987), and some sleep and substance-use disorders. The difficulties often found in separating obsessive-compulsive disorder from other conditions is most common when obsessive compulsive symptoms are secondary symptoms (Pigott *et al.*, 1994). True primary obsessive-compulsive disorder is a clear-cut diagnosis that makes it distinct from anxiety disorders (Montgomery, 1993). When a condition such as alcohol dependence is associated more often with every known psychiatric diagnosis than a control population (Helzer and Pryzbeck, 1988), it is reasonable to suppose that some of these associations may be false ones.

True Association (Secondary)

In these conditions, the comorbidity is in a special form in which anxiety is either a necessary precursor of the other condition or a natural consequence of it. However, because the anxiety is not a fundamental component of the disorder — it is either a trigger or a sequel — the association is not as strong as consanguinity. Winokur (1990) is one of the main proponents for a classification of disorders based on the primary-secondary distinction. This distinction is a long-standing one which was first identified by Munro (1966) and Woodruff and his colleagues (1967) with respect to depression. It was elaborated by Winokur and his colleagues at the University of Iowa Department of Psychiatry long before the advent of DSM-III and may have suffered somewhat by not defining its terms adequately. It also can be criticised because the memories of patients are not always as accurate as we would like, and if the identification of a previous disorder depends entirely on interview it is often subject to error.

Table 9.3 Distinction Between Primary and Secondary Anxiety Disorder (derived in part from Winokur, 1990)

Primary	Secondary
Anxiety disorder is first disorder in chronological sequence	Anxiety is second or later disorder in chronological sequence
Anxiety and the other disorders occur within the space of two years (in any order) and anxiety is the chronic disorder (chemistry is not defined)	Anxiety and the other disorders occur within the space of two years (in any order) and anxiety is **not** the chronic disorder
Anxiety is second disorder in chronological sequence but there is a period of at least two years free of symptoms before anxiety disorder begins	Anxiety is second disorder in chronological sequence but there is a period of less than two years free of symptoms before anxiety disorder begins

The main distinctions between primary and secondary anxiety disorders (derived from Winokur's terminology but adapted for the purposes of anxiety) are shown in Table 9.3. It will be noted immediately that some of the distinctions are arbitrary and become necessary because the simple definition of primary anxiety (a condition which precedes all other psychiatric disorders), can sometimes be defective when there is a long time interval between the two conditions and it is hard to conceive of any clear causal association between them. At the same time, it is important to recognise that there are other disorders in which there is a long time interval between the two disorders in which the association is still a real one, the most obvious being bipolar affective disorder, in which the interval between episodes may be many years but does not in any way affect the diagnosis.

There are many examples of secondary association which are grouped under the general heading of comorbidity and some of the more significant ones not already described elsewhere in this chapter are shown in Table 9.4. The findings illustrate some of the false trails set by comorbidity; their interpretation is open to many different explanations

Table 9.4 Common Forms of Comorbidity Between Anxiety and Other Psychiatric Disorders

Author	Psychiatric Disorders Associated with Anxiety Diagnosis(es)	Degree of Correspondence With Anxiety Disorder	Comments
Simon and VonKorff, 1991	Somatisation disorder	50%	Greater somatisation associated with greater distress and anxiety suggesting somatisation is not a defence against anxiety
Battaglia *et al.*, 1995	Somatisation disorder	25% women, 6% men	Figures applied to panic disorder only; despite these findings disorders considered separate
Brown *et al.*, 1990	Somatisation disorder	34% (GAD) 31% (phobic disorders)	These authors suggest that the figures indicate "a common diathesis"
Haver and Dahlgren, 1995	Alcohol dependence	38%	Mood disorders commonly associated (48%)
Rounsaville *et al.*, 1991	Cocaine abuse	30%	Anxiety disorder usually preceded cocaine abuse; depression followed abuse
George *et al.*, 1990	Alcohol abuse	30%	Anxiety disorder postulated to be cause of panic attacks following alcohol withdrawal
Johnson *et al.*, 1990	Parasuicide (Deliberate self-harm)	7% in patients with panic disorder	Similar association for patients with major depression (7–9%)
Bronisch and Wittchen, 1994	Parasuicide (Deliberate self-harm)	16%	2–4% of total subjects had a self-harm episode
Yonkers, 1997	Premenstrual tension	10%	Anxiety precedes premenstrual symptoms
Sherbourne *et al.*, 1996	Chronic medical condition	10–12% current state	Anxiety is early consequence of chronic disorder
Wells *et al.*, 1989	Chronic medical condition	57% lifetime diagnosis	Anxiety is early consequence of chronic disorder

Table 9.4   (*Continued*)

Author	Psychiatric Disorders Associated with Anxiety Diagnosis(es)	Degree of Correspondence With Anxiety Disorder	Comments
Wessely *et al.*, 1996	Chronic fatigue syndrome (CFS)	30%	Strong correlation between number of symptoms in both CFS and psychiatric disorder
Castillo *et al.*, 1995	Stroke (cerebral haemorrhage/infarction)	27% pre-stroke 23% post-stroke	Early onset of anxiety in those with a previous history of psychiatric disorder
Merikangas and Angst, 1995	Major depression	20% of social phobics	Social phobia precedes onset of major depression — greater handicap if comorbid
Hecht *et al.*, 1989	Depression	40%	Current state — all anxiety disorders included
Ball *et al.*, 1995	Depression	10%	Incidence in panic disorder only
Van Ameringen *et al.*, 1991	Depression	Social phobia 70%	Alcohol abuse (28%); substance abuse (16%). Social phobia precedes other diagnoses
Thompson *et al.*, 1989	Depression	Complex relationship	Comorbidity of panic greater with depression than with agoraphobia; a finding which runs counter to current classification of panic
Barsky *et al.*, 1994 (Similar — Barsky *et al.*, 1992)	Hypochondriasis in primary care	1.6% (panic disorder)	Association is so low that it could be explained by true comorbidity
Braun *et al.*, 1994	Eating disorder	40%	Patients with anorexia more likely to develop eating disorder first
Flick *et al.*, 1993	Personality disorder	40%	Associated with cluster C personality disorders

Table 9.4 (*Continued*)

Author	Psychiatric Disorders Associated with Anxiety Diagnosis(es)	Degree of Correspondence With Anxiety Disorder	Comments
Oldham *et al.*, 1995	Personality disorder	30–50%	Associated with cluster C and borderline personality disorders
Vaglum and Vaglum, 1989	Borderline schizotypal personality	60%	Selected sample of female patients with alcohol dependence
Herbert *et al.*, 1992	Avoidant personality disorder	75% (social phobia)	No evidence that these conditions are separate disorders

NB: All indicate some form of association greater than chance, apart from the studies by Barsky *et al* (1992, 1994) between hypochondriasis and anxiety disorders.

as the evidence available, despite its clean-cut and impeccable appearance, is equivocal.

Somatisation disorder is frequently associated with anxiety disorder, and this will hardly be surprising as it fits one of the main hypotheses expressed in this book, that anxiety expressed mainly in the form of bodily symptoms, which can be called somatosthenic anxiety (Tyrer, 1982), is only the extreme of the anxiety disorder spectrum, and therefore belongs with anxiety. The findings that comorbidity between the two groups is around 50%, with somewhat lesser rates for individual anxiety disorders such as panic and phobias (Table 9.4) only really refutes one hypothesis, that somatisation is a psychodynamic defence against the expression of anxiety (on the grounds that somatisation is the acceptable and anxiety the unacceptable face of anxiety (see Chapter 3)). Even this hypothesis is not fully refuted by the data; it is possible to argue that much of the anxiety symptoms associated with somatisation are secondary features that follow from perception of the somatic symptoms.

Substance use is also highly associated with other mental disorders independent of addiction, with around one in four people with a substance misuse disorder in epidemiological samples having a mental state disorder also (Regier *et al.*, 1990b), although anxiety disorders are not as prominent as some disorders such as bipolar disorders and schizophrenia. In patient samples, the degree of association is higher and the data is not really adequate to argue which comes first, the substance misuse (which then leads to anxiety disorders after addiction and withdrawal symptoms have developed, as George *et al.* (1990) argue); or the anxiety symptoms (particularly social anxiety) which are a precursor to initial drug abuse before dependence and addiction become established (Rounsaville *et al.*, 1991).

Self-harm is less common in anxiety than depression but only when the conditions exist in their (less common) single form. In one study (Bronisch and Wittchen, 1994), cases with pure major depression did not have an odds ratio for suicide attempts significantly higher than subjects with no DSM-III diagnosis, but those with comorbid major depression and a lifetime-anxiety-disorder diagnosis showed significantly elevated odds ratios. This again opens up the debate about the exact nature of the relationship between anxiety and depression. Although the comorbidity studies in Table 9.4 emphasise the high rates of association, they do not indicate its nature. Even the interesting finding that greater comorbidity is found for depression than agoraphobia in the case of panic disorder (Thompson *et al.*, 1989) is not necessarily indicative of any particular relationship between them.

The primary-secondary distinction is of relatively little help in establishing the meaning of comorbidity even though it is possible to place the onset of disorders in a chronological sequence. Some disorders, such as social phobia and anorexia nervosa, begin early in life and so it is not surprising that they are primary in chronological terms. This does not necessarily mean that the first is of special significance in predisposing towards the second, although it is often interpreted in this way (Van Ameringen *et al.*, 1991; Regier *et al.*, 1998).

The association between personality disorder and anxiety disorders is an interesting issue which could be regarded as different from other forms of comorbidity, as the personality domain is separate from the mental state one (at least in the DSM-IV classification) and therefore could be regarded as a co-axial rather than a comorbid diagnosis. The strongest association is between anxiety and the cluster C group of personality disorders (dependent, anxious (avoidant in the DSM-IV classification), and anankastic (obsessive-compulsive in the DSM-IV classification) personality disorders. Here there is usually no argument which condition is the primary one. Personality disorder begins early in life and is manifest by the time of adolescence at the latest. It therefore begins earlier than most anxiety diagnoses, with the possible exception of simple phobias which may originate even earlier.

It is also important to recognise that medical conditions can also give rise to pathological forms of anxiety quite separate from any understandable anxiety that can be created by worry over physical illness. Chronic medical disorders, in particular, can be very commonly associated with anxiety and in such instances, it appears that the medical condition is a necessary precursor and the anxiety disorder is a genuine secondary one.

True Association (Consanguinity)

Are any of the associations already identified sufficiently strong to regard the comorbid conditions as identical or constituting the same condition. Again it is impossible to be certain, and the figures indicating the degree of comorbidity are not of particular value here. It is quite possible that one disorder may have been classified incorrectly and actually consists of two disorders, one which is an integral component of another and the other which is separate. The comorbidity rate could be 50% for the mixed disorder but 100% for that component which is an integral part of the consanguid condition.

The most obvious example of a consanguid condition is mixed anxiety-depression disorder, in which diagnostic criteria have recently been established by a DSM-IV task force and which gives equal weight to anxiety and depressive symptoms. Another example is that of the diagnosis of adjustment disorder with mixed anxiety and depressive symptoms (F43.22 in ICD-10 and 309.28 in DSM-IV), a relatively uncommon diagnosis in ordinary psychiatric practice, but which I have found increasingly useful in my own.

Table 9.5 A Scale for the Diagnosis of the General Neurotic Syndrome

Positive features	Score	Negative features	Score
Simultaneous presence of anxiety and depressive symptoms, each sufficiently severe to qualify for a formal anxiety and depressive diagnosis* and normally lasting for two months or longer	+2	Persistent phobic or obsessional symptoms for three months or longer	-2
At least one change in primacy of anxiety and depressive symptoms at different times in the course of the disorder	+3	Anxiety and depressive symptoms only presenting within one month of major life stresses or events	-3
Co-occurrence of phobic, panic, obsessional or hypochondriacal symptoms of variable severity, but not persisting for longer than three months	+1		
Dependent or anxious (avoidant) premorbid personality disorder*	+3	Antisocial, histrionic, impulsive or borderline personality disorder*	-3
Anankastic (obsessive compulsive) personality disorder*	+1		
At least one first-degree relative has a similar mixed anxiety-depressive disorder	+2		

* Using ICD-10 or DSM-IV criteria.
A score of 4 or more indicates the presence of the syndrome.
(The first negative feature — phobic and obsessional symptoms can be omitted unless it is wished to separate these disorders).

The association between anxiety, depression and cluster C personality disorder has been noted frequently in the literature, and in 1985 I suggested that this condition, the general neurotic syndrome, might represent the core element of neurosis (Tyrer, 1985). The main characteristics of the syndrome are the simultaneous presence of anxiety and depressive disorders, at least one change in the primacy of anxiety and depression at different times, the presence of dependent and/or anankastic (obsessive-compulsive) personality features, and a family history of a similar disorder. This has been incorporated into a scale for the diagnosis of the general neurotic syndrome (GNS) (Table 9.5). Early suggestions that a score of 6 was necessary for the diagnosis have been modified with further analysis of data and a score of 4 is now considered to be the threshold for diagnosis. The criteria in Table 9.3 separate the specific mixed diagnosis from phobic and obsessional disorders but as these two disorders may also exist in conjunction with the general neurotic syndrome the weighted items separating them might not be considered essential.

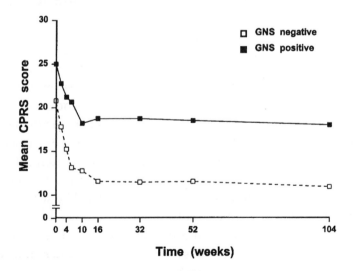

Fig. 9.2 Mean changes in total psychopathology scores using the Comprehensive Psychopathological Rating Scale (CPRS) for patients with the general neurotic syndrome (GNS positive) (n = 66) and those without (GNS negative) (n = 98) in the Nottingham Study of Neurotic Disorder (from Tyrer *et al.*, 1992).

The general neurotic syndrome is postulated as a consanguid condition which is a coaxial one as it covers the domains of personality and mental state disorder (Tyrer et al., 1992). It is supported by data from a range of clinical and genetic studies (Andrews et al., 1990; Angst and Dobler-Mikola, 1991; Tyrer et al., 1991; Larkin et al., 1992). One of the main reasons for identifying it as a separate disorder is the evidence that it has a worse prognosis than other forms of anxiety disorder. This is illustrated in Fig. 9.2, which shows data from the Nottingham Study of Neurotic Disorder. Those who scored positive for the general neurotic syndrome had a significantly worse symptomatic outcome than those without the syndrome after two years (Tyrer et al., 1992) (Fig. 9.2). This difference was even greater after five years, when the presence of the general neurotic syndrome and personality disorder was the best predictor of outcome after age (younger patients had a significantly better outcome than older ones) (Seivewright et al., 1998).

MAKING SENSE OF COMORBIDITY, CO-OCCURRENCE AND ASSOCIATION

Unless I have missed an important element of the construct or in some other way am blind to the obvious, the whole notion of comorbidity seems to be fundamentally a synthetic one which is wrong-headed and counterproductive in research terms. However, associations between disorder exist and cannot be ignored. I think it is possible to make some attempt to separate the different forms of association as described above, but it still involves large elements which are independent of the data obtained. The most common difficulties are with the moderate associations described and illustrated in Table 9.4. The separation into the four types of association discussed above is shown in Fig. 9.3. The arguments over whether the conditions should be conjoined or separated is not in the last resort a useful issue in clinical practice, but whether one of the conditions is a predisposing vulnerability factor or a complication of the other is important and should be investigated. However, it is through other means than massive epidemiological enquiries and other cross-sectional studies that the form of the association

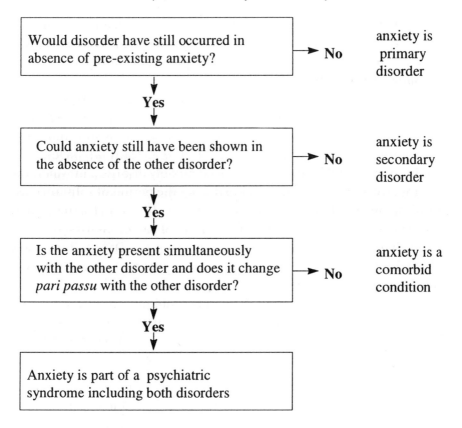

Fig. 9.3 Evaluating the association of anxiety with other disorders.

should be investigated, and these must follow their longitudinal course to some extent.

There are other associations between anxiety and other disorders that are shown in Fig. 9.1 but not described here. The relationship between anxiety and the schizophrenic disorders is one, but the comorbidity literature has nothing of note to say about this important subject. The whole subject of "organic anxiety", anxiety disorders that appear to be similar to others described in this chapter but which are almost certainly caused by brain injury or disease, or sometimes by metabolic abnormalities, is also rarely mentioned. Temporal lobe epilepsy, thyrotoxicosis, phaeochromocytoma (adrenaline-secreting tumours), sarcoidosis, tuberculosis, lupus erythematosus and intermittent acute porphyria can all induce states of panic or more generalised anxiety, which are technically comorbid with the physical disorder if the rules are followed as for other disorders.

The worry about the comorbidity industry is that it responds to repeated findings of strong associations with yet more diagnostic categories, that allow yet more investigations of new associations and new comorbidity findings; where will it end? Already we have a new condition in DSM-IV, substance-induced anxiety disorder, in which the symptoms of anxiety have to develop during the period of substance use or within one month of withdrawal, and which, incidentally, the anxiety may be generalised or obsessive or in the form of panic. It is to be sincerely hoped that wiser counsel will come to bear on the DSM-V Task Force (which doubtless is already meeting in some quiet corner) in such a way that the interminable splitting of diagnosis into smaller and smaller fragments will finally be halted. If anxiety is ubiquitous, it is universally comorbid in one form or another, and the subject needs no further discussion.

Chapter 10

THE CENTRAL CORE OF PATHOLOGICAL ANXIETY

On many occasions in the previous nine chapters I have been critical of current established thinking about the description, classification, treatment and outcome of anxiety disorders. Some may feel, like Don Quixote, that I have been tilting at windmills that are not really fundamental to the concept of anxiety, but I hope I have convinced the reader by this stage that the issues are important ones and that the data from clinical experience and research studies do not bear out most of the hypotheses derived from experimental laboratories or academic institutions that carry out clinical research on a highly selective minority of patients.

In this chapter, however, I have to come clean with some positive replacements for the buildings I have tried to knock down. Before doing this, it is worthwhile listing the structures I have been attacking at various times during the course of this book and for the reader to decide whether they are still standing.

ANXIETY AND DEPRESSION ARE SEPARATE MENTAL DISORDERS

This statement appears to be built on firm foundations as both major classification schemes in psychiatry have anxiety disorders in one major grouping and depressive disorders in a separate one. If one takes this classification as it stands, anxiety and depression are not only in separate buildings but these buildings are placed at opposite ends of the town.

Nevertheless, the arguments against separation are extremely strong. Whilst it is reasonable to argue that anxiety and depression should always be looked for as different *symptoms* (Barlow, 1985, 1987), this does not mean they are different *disorders*. The universally high associations between symptoms of depression and anxiety can be summarised:

> Anxiety and depression
> Teach us one important lesson;
> Though in separation their study pleases
> We must remember they are not diseases.
> And like wind and rain in stormy weather
> These symptoms always appear together.

THERE ARE SPECIFIC TREATMENTS FOR EACH ANXIETY DISORDER

If this statement was true, all current practitioners who treat anxiety disorders could be indicted. Thus, just as knowledge that someone is receiving vitamin B12 injections must necessarily mean that the diagnosis is that of pernicious anaemia, the description of the treatment should indicate the specific anxiety diagnosis. Of course, this is not the case, as we have abundant evidence that some treatments are effective across the full range of anxiety disorders, and indeed depressive ones.

Nevertheless, it is fair to acknowledge that there are some forms of anxiety in which treatment is clearly linked to the diagnosis (Table 10.1). Anxiety, which is a direct consequence of major life events, particularly if these are unexpected, is treated by a range of psychological treatments — counselling, debriefing, abreaction — which helps to promote adjustment to the event and restore harmony in the person's relationship to the environment. Similarly, when anxiety becomes clearly linked to specific situations, it changes its nature considerably because it is accompanied by avoidance. Prevention of avoidance, linked with direct treatment of anxiety and fear, is the essential focus of the treatment of phobias. Linked to this is the anxiety associated with obsessional disorders in which response prevention, or the promotion of avoidance, is the immediate cause of anxiety, and which becomes the main focus of

Table 10.1 Matching Treatment to Diagnosis in Anxiety Disorders

Nature of Anxiety	Focus of Treatment	Main Disorders
Consequence of major life events	Adjustment	Stress Adjustment disorders
Unfocused and unpredictable	Alleviation of symptoms	Generalised anxiety and panic disorder
Situational anxiety	Prevention of avoidance	Phobias
Illness anxiety	Explanation of symptoms	Somatoform disorders

treatment. The most common form of treatment is the alleviation of symptoms but this should only become the focus when these are unfocused and unpredictable; all too often it is easy not to ask about the source of symptoms and automatically assume that they alone need to be treated.

A third group of anxiety symptoms which are linked to treatment are concerned with illness. As might be expected, most of the symptoms for anxiety in these disorders are bodily ones and are interpreted as those of illness rather than of psychological distress. These include many of the conditions classified under the somatoform disorders, of which hypochondriasis is the most clear cut. Although the focus of treatment is far from clear in this group of disorders, it is essential for the sufferer to find another explanation for his or her symptoms apart from that of physical disease.

Apart from these important exceptions, there is no evidence that any treatment is specific to other forms of anxiety. Most anxiety consists of a group of psychological and somatic symptoms, occurring at different levels of intensity at different times, which causes distress that is usually proportional to the intensity of the symptoms. For these disorders, which may cover generalised anxiety, panic, dysthymic and mixed anxiety-depressive disorders, almost all the treatment available for anxiety could be given at one time or another and there is no clear first-line treatment from the evidence available. In particular, "pharmacological dissection" has failed to identify distinct disorders and psychological dissection has been equally unsuccessful.

ANXIETY COMORBIDITY IS A USEFUL DIAGNOSTIC CONCEPT

Comorbidity for anxiety disorders has been a major subject of investigation ever since the introduction of the DSM-III classification. When it was found that very few anxiety disorders existed in pure form, the right decision should have been to abandon the classification as a failure. Instead, the spurious notion was developed that anxiety comorbidity was a new and exciting concept pregnant with meaning. Although this has been of some value inasmuch as any form of comorbidity is associated with a poorer clinical outcome, this finding is really an expression of the poverty of the DSM-III classification, which almost immediately had to be revised to allow other conditions to be described with anxiety rather than accepting a system in which panic disorder, for example, "trumped" all other neurotic conditions which were considered to be subsumed under it.

Unfortunately, as has been shown in the previous chapter, the study of comorbidity has almost become a scientific discipline in its own right. All over the world keen young researchers, anxious to cut their teeth by making their first contribution to the literature, are encouraged to pick on an easy subject such as comorbidity. Simple cross-sectional studies can yield masses of diagnostic information and, with the help of a few statistical packages, hey presto, we have a paper with lots of original data, covering associations and probabilities, which no journal aspiring to scientific credibility can ignore. My reaction, on reading most such articles on anxiety and its associated disorders, is the same as that of William James a century ago, "I may have been too surfeited by too much reading of classic works of the subject, but I should as lief read verbal descriptions of the shapes of rocks on a New Hampshire farm as toil through them again. They give one nowhere a central point of view, or a deductive or generative principle" (James, 1891). Unless new information comes to light which alters our views substantially, the study of comorbidity in cross-sectional studies should be relegated to the history of diagnosis in psychiatry, an aberrant period when the ability to collate and organise data far surpassed our ability to interpret it.

NORMAL AND PATHOLOGICAL ANXIETY

In defining the core of anxiety disorders, we need clear boundary lines between normal and pathological anxiety on one hand, and the different types of pathological anxiety on the other. The boundary between normal and pathological anxiety is relatively straightforward to identify. We know that anxiety is a valuable emotion that adds spice to our lives and is protective of the species. It is only when the symptoms cause distress and lead to impairment of function that anxiety becomes a problem. This boundary is not determined by a physiological test or the identification of a particular group of symptoms; it is decided by the sufferer, and this is how it should be.

The separation of pathological anxiety into smaller groups is a little more problematical. Sigmund Freud, as noted in Chapter 3, described "normal anxiety is anxiety about a real danger", whereas "neurotic anxiety is anxiety about a danger that is yet to be discovered" (Freud, 1926). The presence of real danger conveniently separates the two types of pathological anxiety (Table 10.2). Anxiety that is understandable, and by this I mean understandable to an external observer as well as to the sufferer, can be severe and distressing, not only before the danger is expected but also after a dangerous event. Most stress and adjustment disorders come into this category. All other types of pathological anxiety are inexplicable in that, although the sufferer may have some notion in what way the anxiety has come about, most external observers would not be able to understand it. This even includes some forms of post-traumatic stress disorder, as these can occur long after a stressful event and the reasons for their manifestations are apparently fickle and capricious.

Table 10.2 The Two Main Types of Pathological Anxiety

Type	Features	Diagnostic groups
Understandable pathological anxiety	Anxiety about a real danger, either experienced or expected	Stress and adjustment disorders (including most post-traumatic stress disorders)
Inexplicable pathological anxiety	Anxiety without clear evidence of danger	All other anxiety diagnoses (and some post-traumatic stress disorders)

THE SIGNIFICANCE OF SYMPTOMS IN PATHOLOGICAL ANXIETY

Typical anxiety includes both bodily (somatic) and psychological symptoms and there is no point in repeating these again here. However, we should also appreciate that the extent to which psychological or bodily symptoms are shown varies greatly in different forms of anxiety and this is summarised in Fig. 10.1. The existing systems of justification are atheoretical and therefore give no clue as to why some anxiety disorders present primarily in the somatic sphere and others with psychological features being paramount or with equal psychological and somatic symptoms.

Threat can be used in helping to understand the different diagnoses of anxiety. This is based on the premise that all anxiety is a consequence of response to threat and it is the way in which the threat is received and interpreted that determines the diagnostic form of the anxiety. As noted in Chapter 7, anxiety can be generated without any conscious awareness of an anxiety-provoking stimulus. This "limbic" recognition of threat leads to conventional symptoms of anxiety but, because there is no obvious reason for the anxiety, the symptoms can be interpreted in many different ways. However, in most instances there are conventional feelings of anxiety, with a combination of psychological distress and physical symptoms that is best described as generalised anxiety. This anxiety is

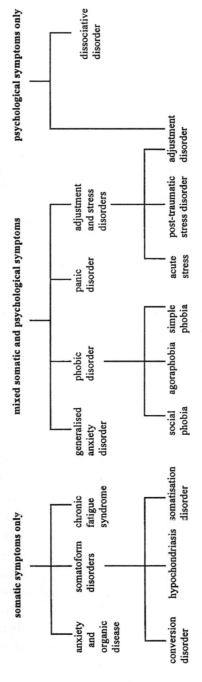

Fig. 10.1 Classification of anxiety symptoms into current diagnostic categories (ICD-10).

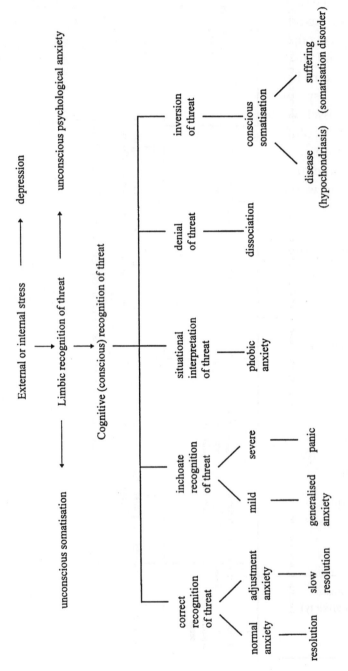

Fig. 10.2 Dynamic flow chart of anxiety and its symptoms.

genuinely "free-floating"; it has nothing to attach itself to because the source of the anxiety has not been identified in consciousness. However, if there is preoccupation over one or more of the symptoms, they can be magnified and distorted so that either one or more psychological or bodily symptoms become overvalued in terms of its significance.

The initial symptoms following the perception of threat include a mixture of psychological and bodily symptoms, such as that shown in the left-hand column of Table 10.3. Following feedback from these symptoms, and consequent preoccupation with one or more of them, the order of hierarchy changes. The example shown in Table 10.3 comes from a young woman whose mother had been recently diagnosed as

Table 10.3 How Over-valued Symptoms Can Lead to Diagnostic Shift

Hierarchy of Anxiety Symptoms		
Feeling anxious	Feeling anxious	**Feeling dizzy**
Cannot concentrate	Cannot concentrate	Muscle cramps
Panicky	Muscle cramps	Palpitaions
Palpitations	**Feeling dizzy**	Muscle tension
Muscle tension	Palpitations	Feeling anxious
Muscle cramps	Panicky	Cannot concentrate
Sleep disturbance	Muscle tension	Panicky
Feeling dizzy	Sleep disturbance	Sleep disturbance
Restlessness	Restlessness	Restlessness
Initial symptoms (Generalised anxiety)	Consequences of over-valuation (somatisation)	Consequences of over-valuation (hypochondriacal disorder)

having multiple sclerosis. When the symptoms of anxiety, possibly created at least partly by her mother's illness, were first shown, the feeling of dizziness was relatively low in the hierarchy. However, because this struck a chord with her mother's initial symptoms of multiple sclerosis, the value attached to dizziness became more and more pronounced so that by the time of referral to a psychiatrist, it had become the most dominant symptom. At this stage, she was diagnosed as having a hypochondriacal disorder but examination of the precursors of the condition showed that it was initially a straightforward, simple anxiety diagnosis.

RELATIONSHIP BETWEEN ANXIETY AND DEPRESSION

Although depression, and its counterpart, mania, have appropriated for themselves the title of "mood disorders" in current diagnostic classifications, it is important to be reminded that anxiety is also a mood. The two moods are intimately associated, so that whenever one alters the other does to some extent as well. This is seen in its most marked form in adjustment reactions to major stresses and in the emotionally unstable personality disorders, impulsive and borderline conditions. In these conditions, depression and anxiety can predominate at different times but changeover is so fast and frequent, the mood is described as labile. It takes only the slightest stimulus to change the person from intense, anxious preoccupation to the depths of despair and sometimes a change can occur even without any apparent stimulus. Although it is conventional to regard this type of mood change as quite different from mood variations in anxiety and depression, the differences are only ones of degree.

In any anxious or depressive disorder, whatever emotion is demonstrated on the surface is only part of the story. The alternative emotion, anxiety or depression, is present beneath the surface and can be detected by clinical interview, even if only assessed crudely and simply. For the mild disorders, it is easier to identify both emotions because there is less disorder to examine and the whole can be seen much more easily than when the disorder gets more severe. In the most extreme cases, such as depressive stupor, the external appearance is totally of

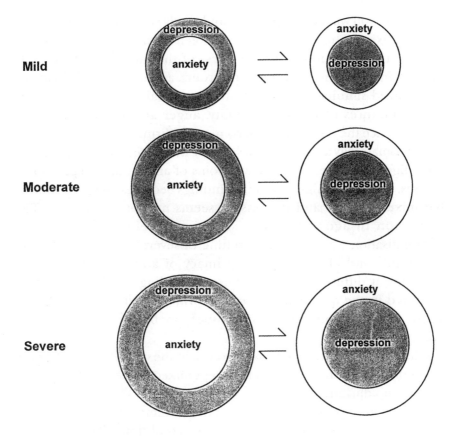

Fig. 10.3 Relationship between anxiety and depression.

one emotion. However, even here, there is intense anxiety underneath and this is often only elicited after the sufferer has improved and can talk about their innermost feelings when they have been unwell (Fig. 10.3).

In more severe depression and anxiety the range and depth of symptoms become greater and, at the extremes of the range, it is possible to identify what appears to be "pure" anxiety or depressive disorders. Unfortunately, this perception is wrong and illustrates all the disadvantages of a simple atheoretical classification of psychiatric disorders based on the expression of symptoms only. Dig deep into anxiety and you will find depression and similar digging into depression will find anxiety. The only difference between the milder and more severe forms of the condition is the thickness of the outer layer (Fig. 10.3). Whereas in stress and adjustment disorders, anxiety and depression are experienced simultaneously and often in equal proportion, together with admixtures of panic, irritability, anger and social behavioural changes, once the disorder has become more firmly based, several layers of symptomatology and behaviour become integrated into the condition. The diligent observer will find symptoms of anxiety and depression in all cases, but the terminology of the findings becomes changed subtly so that mixed anxiety and depression seems no longer to exist. Thus depression in agoraphobia according to Klein (1981) becomes "demoralisation"; anxiety in the setting of severe depression becomes "agitation"; and changes in the primacy of anxiety and depressive symptoms at different times becomes, according to Winokur (1990), enshrined in the qualifying adjectives "primary and secondary" which are given special significance in diagnostic terms but are limited in clinical utility.

What is so curious about those involved in the classification of anxiety and depression is the readiness to accept mixed anxiety and depressive features in adjustment and stress disorders and in the "sub-threshold" mixed anxiety-depressive disorder, but the extreme reluctance to extend this combined diagnosis to more severe conditions. These are only quantitative variations of the minor disorders, so the refusal to acknowledge the combination of anxiety and depression in these disorders is difficult to justify on any rational basis.

The acceptance of mixed anxiety-depressive disorders at all levels of severity of affective disturbance does not mean that the presenting symptoms should be ignored. As Fig. 10.3 indicates for each level of severity, there is a range between the dominant expression of anxiety symptoms and a similar expression of symptoms of depression. As described earlier in the account of the Nottingham Study of Neurotic Disorder, in the short- and medium terms those who present originally with anxiety symptoms tend to continue to present them and, similarly, those already presenting with symptoms of depression continue with more depressive symptoms than anxiety ones. In the longer term, however, the opposite affect forces itself into full consciousness and behaviour, and no clinician should be surprised that after an interval of many years, it is impossible to discover any relationship between the presenting condition and that which occurred in the first episode.

LIFE EVENTS AND ANXIETY

Life events are a major source of external threat and therefore are essential to the study of clinical anxiety. With this in mind, it is perhaps surprising that there have not been more studies to examine the effect of life events in anxiety disorders, particularly as relationship between life events and almost every other psychiatric disorder, as well as many physical ones, have been examined in such depth.

The most important fact in this subject to be remembered is that life events in approximately 90% of people, despite their apparent severity, create no demonstrable symptoms in people exposed to them. In Shakespeare's panegyric to the qualities of our species, "what a piece of work is man, how noble in reason, how infinite in faculty, in form, in moving how express and admirable" could well have been added "how resilient in adversity". It is perhaps natural in studies of morbidity to look at vulnerability rather than resilience, but the latter does repay attention, as Rutter (1985) has emphasised. The factors that lead to vulnerability in response to life events, with consequence exhibition of anxiety and other neurotic symptoms, are many but, as has been indicated earlier, pre-morbid personality appears to be the most fundamental. Although personality status appears little in the voluminous literature on life events and authors such as Brown and Harris (1978, 1993) repeatedly refer to "vulnerability factors" such as loss of a parent, the number of children in the family, absence of earned income and others in listing these; many of these factors are not only related to personality but are a direct consequence of it. If it was therefore possible to assess personality status reliably and validly, this would be of immense benefit in determining who responds badly to life events and in what way. In the last 30 years, there has been a general feeling amongst most social scientists that personality cannot be assessed adequately for this purpose.

This was seen at its most extreme in the 1960s and 70s in which the whole notion of individual personalities that persisted for long periods came under intense criticism (Mischel, 1973). Unfortunately, most of the work leading to this conclusion was carried out in young university students at times in their lives when adaptation to change was most important. The results, therefore, suggested that personality shifted a great deal, whereas it is much more likely (in retrospect) that the changes observed were those associated with adapting to changing environments rather than a fundamental change in core personality.

The major distinction between normal personality and personality disorder, or, more accurately, across the personality continuum between normal personality, personality difficulty, single and diffuse personality disorder (Tyrer and Johnson, 1996) the increasing lack of ability to adapt to circumstances as personality disorder becomes more pronounced. In other words, normal personality becomes personality disorder when it ceases to adapt to circumstances. The classification of personality disorder has been far from satisfactory and has led to a great deal of argument since formal classifications became of age in 1980 with the introduction of the third edition of the *Diagnostic and Statistical Manual for Mental Disorders* (DSM-III) (American Psychiatric Association, 1980), and this has not been adequately resolved (and may be one of the main reasons why many workers disregard personality disorder as an appropriate subject for study). Personality disorder still retains an aura of diagnostic unacceptability. The other somewhat unsatisfactory inference of the diagnosis of personality disorder is that, by definition, it is an enduring condition that begins in adolescence and persists for long periods in life (although not indefinitely as was originally thought), and therefore it invokes all the ideas of predestination and inevitability that made Freudian theory so unpopular. Its implication that social forces have very little to play in the outcome and development of the disorder, is also profoundly dissatisfying in our current "age of empowerment" in which all handicaps have the potential to be overcome.

In fact we now have a very much better notion of personality disorder than we did 20 years ago. Our notion of it is far from satisfactory in developmental terms (Rutter, 1987), but our descriptions have become more reliable and cross-national studies have established that the criteria for definition are robust (Tyrer *et al.*, 1984; Loranger *et al.*, 1994). Personality disorder can now describe itself in the same way as Groucho Marx defined himself, "I have been raised from nothing to a state of absolute poverty". However, even strong critics of the definition and classification of personality disorder, of whom I am one, acknowledge that the attempts to formulate the classification and description of personality disorder, despite their imperfections, are a definite improvement on what has gone before (Tyrer, 1995).

The hypothesis put forward here is that personality disorder is the key factor creating vulnerability to life events so that the individual concerned appears emotionally unstable and overreacts to events to the extent that they develop a neurotic disorder in one or more of its many forms (Fig. 10.4). The individual with personality disorder reacts in various ways to try and reduce the impact of life events, such as over-investing in relationships with one or two individuals or avoiding unpredictable life events by gross restriction of life style, but these are essentially maladaptive and are liable to break down. An important corollary of the hypothesis is that breakdown creates life events of its own and so the cycle of vulnerability is reinforced (Fig. 10.4). Life for the personality disordered patient is one long set of adjustment disorders

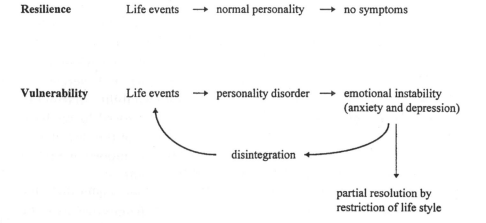

Fig. 10.4 Life events, personality and anxiety.

Table 10.4 How Personality Disorder Creates Vulnerability to Life Events

Stage	Main feature	Characteristics
Stage 1	Personality development	Absence of security and stable attachment in early years
Stage 2	Distortion of help-support systems	Difficulty or inability to draw on appropriate support at times of distress
Stage 3	Shift to external locus of control	Failure to develop internal systems of monitoring and determining attitudes and behaviour so person is constantly reacting to events
Stage 4	Absence of defences against adversity	Inability to adapt to changes so minor events become major catastrophes

in which adjustment to each event is never achieved but supplanted by yet another new event.

It may be useful to consider how personality disorder alters the ability of the individual to cope satisfactorily with life events. This can be examined in developmental terms and is illustrated in Table 10.4. Before personality has developed to any significant degree, a child is much more susceptible to the effect of life events although, even at this young age, the effects of temperament, the precursor of personality, may be considerable (Rutter, 1987) and can be identified within the first two years of life (Kagan *et al.*, 1978). In the presence of favourable conditions for personality development, which appear to involve secure and stable attachments in the early years of life, the individual develops a degree of resilience and autonomy that helps to cope with adversity.

This ability also includes the prudent use of support from others at a time of particular difficulty; by a process of trial and error, the growing child learns gradually to fine tune requests for help and to learn the limitations and scope of his or her own personal resources. By this stage the person prone to personality disorder is already at a significant disadvantage. The limits of personal resourcefulness have not been properly tested, there are few appropriate supporters to draw on at times of distress, and the positive aspects of trial and error become replaced by random access to a variety of, largely inappropriate, support figures. Thus children with conduct disorder, which so often develops into antisocial personality disorder in adult life, derive much of their support from their peers with conduct disorder and achieve their individual identity by investing their personality in groups or gangs. Similarly, those with passive and dependent personality characteristics become excessively reliant on a small number of people and indulge in excessive help-seeking.

In the next stage of development, those destined to remain free of personality disorder develop a clear notion of themselves as autonomous individuals who are able to exercise control of events and determine their own destinies. Those who are well on the way to becoming personality disordered do not have this autonomy, have not learned from experience, and have little reserves to draw on when encountering the unexpected. This difference has been well described by Rotter (1966) in terms of "locus of control". A person with an internal locus of control is confident and secure, with the expectation that any changes that take place are likely to be determined by their own efforts rather than by chance events, and only needs to draw the help of others at times of crisis. Those with an external locus of control seem to have lives that are dictated by events and for which they take no responsibility. Thus there is always someone, or something, else to blame for their misfortunes.

The final stage of personality development is achieved in early adult life with the construction of defences against adversity, particularly unexpected adversity. Many of these defences are developed to prevent the inappropriate expression of emotions such as anger, depression, anxiety and irritability. More complex defences help to put unpleasant subjects that cause distress in the back rooms of consciousness so that they do not interfere too much with daily functioning. Although defences are often considered in psychoanalytical teachings to be counterproductive and maladaptive, they all have a part to play in the normal mechanisms of dealing with adversity.

The defences adopted by those with personality disorders are of a much more primitive and less helpful kind. They involve the classic mechanisms of projection (others are to blame for my troubles and I would be perfectly well if they had not treated me this way), and introjection (no one else in the world can be trusted, so "you have to look after number one"). There is always an external explanation for misfortunes in which case the person avoids taking responsibility for their own actions or responses to events (Tyrer, 1999).

The overall consequence of this primitive and confrontational behaviour is that life events, whether created by the personality abnormality or occurring independently, are perceived as unstoppable and inevitable and blown up out of all proportion to their significance. Thus, for example, a minor event such as a close relative going away for a holiday abroad, can be interpreted as a punishing rejection motivated by personal malice. This is then followed by a gamut of emotions — anger, guilt, depression and anxiety — that can lead to behaviour that creates its own life events (e.g. self-harm, aggression). This tendency is well demonstrated in those with a flamboyant or dramatic group of personality disorders which have higher rates of life events than other personalities (Seivewright, 1987; Torgersen *et al.*, 1998, to be published).

INTERNAL REINFORCEMENT OF ANXIETY

Because anxiety is such an important element of normal human existence that serves a variety of positive functions, it is quite inappropriate to attempt to quell it entirely. The life of an anxiety-free society is well described in Aldous Huxley's book, *Brave New World*, in which all people receive a "happy pill", soma, as part of their regular diet and thereby no longer experience anxiety symptoms. Anxiety only becomes handicapping when it arises inappropriately and persists when there is no real threat still present.

Life events are external precipitants of anxiety but we should not forget that the symptoms of anxiety themselves can be equally instrumental in reinforcing anxiety. Both the psychological and somatic

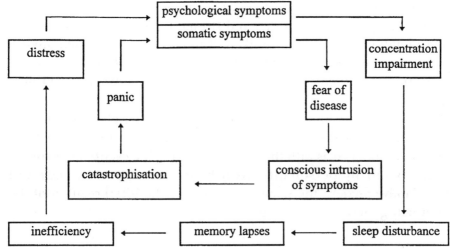

Fig. 10.5 Reinforcers of somatic and psychological anxiety.

symptoms of anxiety can act as reinforcers and therefore cause anxiety to persist long after it should have disappeared (Fig. 10.5).

Anxiety symptoms are potent reinforcers because they can promote the feelings of uncertainty that are central to the core of anxiety. The sensation of threat and problems in concentration caused by anxiety prevents tasks from being carried out and the cycle of inefficiency, sleep disturbance, inability to remember things that one can normally remember, and the distress created by all these feelings, is extreme anxiety provoking in itself. In addition, if the symptoms become overvalued, they can create whole new systems of anxiety in their own right. A great deal of insomnia is the consequence of temporary anxiety associated with insomnia, followed by anxiety-about-insomnia, leading to "learned insomnia" (i.e. this is my bedroom where I do not sleep; I will therefore stay awake here).

The somatic symptoms of anxiety are even more potent reinforcers because they can simulate a variety of other conditions, particularly organic disease. The ultimate anxiety is a threat to one's continued existence and there are many opportunities in interpreting the physical symptoms of anxiety to come to this conclusion. When the symptoms of anxiety are particularly sudden and strong, for example in panic, this interpretation is all the more likely. The consequence is that anxiety begets anxiety and feedback loops are developed (Fig. 10.5) which are extremely difficult to interrupt once they have become established firmly.

It can therefore be seen that it is not the symptoms of anxiety that are the main problem in the central core of the condition, but their interpretation. Just as with the interpretation of life events, mediated to some extent by personality disturbance, creates consistent and maladaptive anxiety, the same also is true of the interpretation of the internally generated symptoms.

TREATMENT OF ESSENTIAL ANXIETY

We now have a clear notion of the differences between the central core of anxiety and the peripheral aspects that are much less significant in clinical terms. The central core, which can best be termed *essential anxiety*, is anxiety that has become self-reinforcing, either through excessive sensitivity to life events or to misinterpretation of anxiety symptoms. It leads to continual, and sometimes constant, preoccupation with symptoms, general impairment of function and inefficiency. It is also prone to lead to more serious disorder, including the development of phobias and all the handicaps of avoidance, the use of inappropriate treatments such as alcohol as a form of symptom relief, and the development of additional disorders such as hypochondriasis and neurasthenia, which create yet more suffering for the individual. Most essential anxiety is the inexplicable pathological anxiety of Table 10.2; most of the understandable anxieties have not developed to this stage.

Unlike the current classifications of anxiety, which measure severity almost entirely by intensity and nature of symptoms, I argue that essential anxiety requires assessment of the precipitants of symptoms, the way they are interpreted, and the degree to which they impair function, as well as the symptoms themselves (Table 10.5). If, after assessment, essential anxiety is identified through all four of these characteristics

Table 10.5 Characteristics of Essential Anxiety

Attribute	Description
Self-reinforcement	Continued anxiety in the absence of obvious threat
Helplessness	Feeling that anxiety symptoms are outside any form of personal control
Impairment	Both of function and by evoking significant distress (so the individual functions at less than 60% of optimal norm)
Maladaptive responses	Often seen as complications of anxiety but which are mainly inappropriate responses to it (e.g. excessive use of alcohol, frequent medical consultations and treatments, detrimental alteration in life style).

being present that the clinician knows that the anxiety is unlikely to resolve spontaneously and the policy of "wait and see" is out of the question.

TREATMENT OF ESSENTIAL ANXIETY

The decision how to treat anxiety remains a controversial one. In my personal practice, I feel it best in our present state of knowledge to put the options to the patient so that their opinions are taken into account before a final decision is made. This might be regarded as a politically correct nod in the direction of "consumerism", but it is prudent because it is more likely to lead to a therapeutic alliance that will aid compliance with treatment and subsequent resolution.

In deciding whether or not to choose drug treatment, it is important for the clinician to consider all aspects of treatment: initial prescription, maintenance therapy and withdrawal (Fig. 10.6). The last part of this process, the period after reducing and stopping the drug, is perhaps the most important one. Unfortunately, as has been noted many times in earlier in this book, withdrawal problems are often confused with anxiety symptoms and it is impossible to be absolutely certain whether a complex

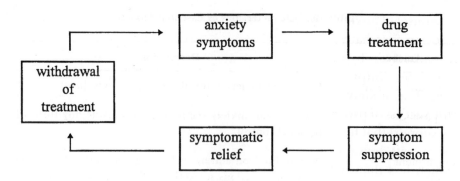

Fig. 10.6 Drug treatment of anxiety.

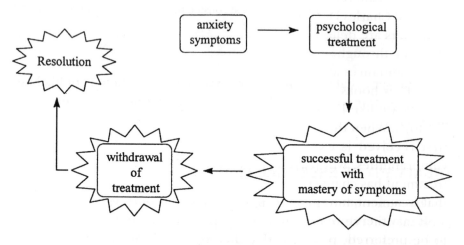

Fig. 10.7 Successful psychological treatment of anxiety.

of symptoms is that of anxiety or that of withdrawal. Unfortunately, even if the symptoms occurring after withdrawal are not related in any way to previous dependence on the drug, they will still be interpreted negatively and the individual will feel that his or her anxiety is returning and therefore treatment needs to be reinstituted.

The real problem with drug treatment is that it does not give the patient any additional resources to cope with anxiety and, when the drug is withdrawn, the patient is just as vulnerable as he was before the onset of anxiety symptoms and prone to react in the same way if they reoccur for whatever reason. With most of the psychological treatments for anxiety — hypnosis is the main exception — the treatment not only alleviates symptoms but also reinforces the patient with methods of repelling anxiety in the future. This is illustrated in Fig. 10.7, in which the success of psychological treatment is accompanied by an extra shield of support that helps to keep further symptoms at bay. As a consequence, when withdrawal of treatment takes place, the likelihood of relapse is much less than with drug treatment. The patient is left with greater strengths and confidence and has a set of strategies for any return of anxiety. In comparing the efficacy of drug and psychological treatment in anxiety, I am reminded of George Orwell's incisive comparison of the merits of Charles Dickens and Nicholas Tolstoy. Whereas all of Dickens' characters are delightfully and often brilliantly portrayed they remain the same throughout his books, whereas Tolstoy's develop in response to circumstances and events and are often very different people at the end of his books than they are at the beginning. Drug treatments in anxiety are like Dickens' characters; psychological treatments are like Tolstoy's. When the drug therapy is withdrawn the same individual who first received is exposed and is subject to all his or her earlier vulnerabilities, whereas the person who has received psychological treatment has changed, sometimes imperceptibly, as a consequence of that treatment and is better buttressed against adversity.

It may therefore be concluded that psychological treatment is much to be preferred to drug treatment and therefore drug treatment, in general, should be phased out. This would be a grave mistake, partly because some people find it extremely difficult to master the psychological treatments available for anxiety or are unresponsive to them. The two modes of treatment are different but not mutually exclusive so that at various times they can be taken independently or combined together.

Normal anxiety is to be expected and has intrinsic value but pathological anxiety, particularly essential anxiety described above, has no useful function. The pragmatic approach, whereby all effective treatments for this group of disorders should be considered when contemplating treatment, is by far the best one. Despite the fact that anxiety is often subsumed within the more dramatic presentations of mental symptomatology, it remains at the heart of most psychotic disorders, and certainly for those described as neurotic. Clinical anxiety is like a slow burning fuse leading to an explosives dump; it may just appear to be in the background for much of the time, but if it is not suppressed or extinguished, there is a danger of massive disintegration. Living with anxiety is not the same as coping with anxiety; and any interventions that we have available to promote coping should always be on hand.

Gray (1982) referred to anxiety as "the Janus continent of mind and brain" with its different faces exposed to the world. This chapter too is concerned with two Janus faces of anxiety; one of normal anxiety, opened and exposed, fully aware of impending dangers and their significance; the other pathological anxiety, cowering in terror of fears it cannot fathom, and magnifying dangers out of all proportion because it knows not what they are. It is this pathological anxiety that is at the core of clinical practice and whether it deposits itself in the acute episodes of panic, the recurring torture of bodily symptoms, the irrationality of phobic fear or the long drawn out agony of generalised anxiety, is not of prime importance; it is the anxiety itself that needs to be tamed, not the diagnosis.

In the final analysis, it is the extent to which pathological anxiety can be controlled that determines whether they persist or not. "I still get my panics, but I don't care about them so they are no longer panics", which is how one patient put this to me. So it is only when anxiety no longer threatens the integrity of the individual that it ceases to be pathological. When normal people receive injections of adrenaline or other sympathomimetic amines, they appear to be anxious and show all the bodily symptoms of people who are anxious, but on questioning they describe the feeling "as if" they had been anxious rather than necessarily experiencing a real anxiety itself. Anxious symptoms are not dysfunctional unless they threaten the integrity of the individual. Sometimes this can be a hangover from normal anxiety, as for example in post-traumatic stress disorder but, more commonly, it seems to become a problem only when tapping into certain vulnerable characteristics of the individual, characteristics which create an Achilles heel and allows the anxiety to get under the protective skin and wreak havoc by spreading uncertainty in all directions.

Prophylaxis against recurrent anxiety can be achieved with drug treatment; most anti-anxiety drugs and anti-depressants, by radical reappraisal of thinking, as in cognitive therapy, and by behavioural approaches, and it is fair to add that they may sometimes occur spontaneously. It is unlikely that this improvement can be measured directly in the central nervous system using current methods of investigation and to date no measure of anxiety has been able to distinguish the expressions of these two different forms of anxiety. At this stage we cannot say whether it is better to reduce the impact of anxiety by treatment with drugs, or by altering the reaction to anxiety so that it is no longer perceived as threatening and unpleasant but rather ignored in the disinterested way one brushes away an aggravating fly. The biological psychiatrists would probably go for the former; those that favour the psychotherapies and cognitive therapy would go for the latter. What is clear is a persistent pathological anxiety of whatever type cannot be conveniently ignored and assumed to get better on its own. "Something has to be done" commented the Prince of Wales (later Edward VIII), seeing the plight of the unemployed in the early 1930s, and although his own contribution was ineffective, he was making a correct protest against the awful consequences of unemployment on the human psyche as well as on the purse. Pathological anxiety should not be unattended because it not only causes suffering in itself, but creates distress for the future when allowed to proceed unchecked. The bringing of such anxiety under control, therefore, serves a double purpose: treatment and future prevention. For normal anxiety, this is not important.

Absence of treatment is probably an advantage as resolution will occur naturally without the unnecessary attribution to a specific intervention. What is necessary for all clinicians to do is to be able to recognise the second Janus face of pathological anxiety whenever it shows the essential core features described in this chapter, so that early intervention can be given before the tendency for mutual reinforcement has become established and the awful feeling of recurring threat is not allowed to haunt our waking lives.

REFERENCES

Adler, R., Hayes, M., Nolan, M., Lewin, T., & Raphael, B. (1991). Antenatal prediction of mother-infant difficulties. *Child Abuse and Neglect*, **15**, 351–361.

Agras, W.S., Sylvester, D., & Oliveau, D.C. (1969). The epidemiology of common fears and phobias. *Comprehensive Psychiatry*, **10**, 151–156.

Akiskal, H.S. (1983). Dysthymic disorder: psychopathology of proposed chronic depressive subtypes. *American Journal of Psychiatry*, **140**, 11–20.

Albus, M., & Scheibe, G. (1993). Outcome of panic disorder with or without concomitant depression: a 2-year prospective follow-up study. *American Journal of Psychiatry*, **150**, 1878–1880.

Alexander, F. (1930). The neurotic character. *International Journal of Psychoanalysis*, **11**, 291–311.

American Psychiatric Association (1980). *Diagnostic and Statistical Manual of Mental Disorders, 3rd revision*. Washington: American Psychiatric Association.

American Psychiatric Association (1994). *Diagnostic and Statistical Manual of Mental Disorders, 4th revision*. Washington: American Psychiatric Association.

Anderson, D.J., Noyes, R.J., & Crowe, R.R. (1984). A comparison of panic disorder and generalized anxiety disorder. *American Journal of Psychiatry*, **141**, 572–575.

Andrews, G. (1990). The diagnosis and management of pathological anxiety. *Medical Journal of Australia*, **152**, 656–659.

Andrews, G., Stewart, G., Morris-Yates, A., Holt, P., & Henderson, S. (1990). Evidence for a general neurotic syndrome. *British Journal of Psychiatry*, **157**, 6–12.

Angst, J., & Dobler-Mikola, A. (1985). The Zurich study: a continuum from depressive to anxiety disorders. *European Archives of Psychiatry and Neurological Sciences*, **235**, 179–186.

Aranko, K., Mattila, M.J., Nuutila, A., & Pellinen, J. (1985). Benzodiazepines, but not antidepressants or neuroleptics, induce dose-dependent development of tolerance to lorazepam in psychiatric patients. *Acta Psychiatrica Scandinavica*, **72**, 436–446.

Armitage, P. (1960). *Sequential Medical Trials*. Oxford: Oxford University Press.

Åsberg, M., Montgomery, S.A., Perris, C., Schalling, D., & Sedvall, G. (1978). A comprehensive psychopathological rating scale. *Acta Psychiatrica Scandinavica* (*Suppl 271*), 5–29.

Asher, R. (1951). Münchausen's syndrome. *Lancet*, **i**, 339–341.

Ashton, C.H., Rawlins, M.D., & Tyrer, S.P. (1990). A double-blind placebo-controlled study of buspirone in diazepam withdrawal in chronic benzodiazepine users. *British Journal of Psychiatry*, **157**, 232–238.

Ashton, H. (1984). Benzodiazepine withdrawal: an unfinished story. *British Medical Journal*, **288**, 1135–1140.

Ashton, H. (1987). Benzodiazepine withdrawal: outcome in 50 patients. *British Journal of Addiction*, **82**, 665–671.

Baker, B.L., Cohen, D.C., & Saunders, J.T. (1973). Self-directed desensitization for acrophobia. *Behavior Research and Therapy*, **11**, 79–89.

Baker, R. (1989). Where does "panic disorder" come from? In: *Panic Disorder: Theory, Research and Therapy* (ed. Baker, R.), p. 9. Chichester: John Wiley.

Ball, S.G., Buchwald, A.M., Waddell, M.T., & Shekhar, A. (1995). Depression and generalized anxiety symptoms in panic disorder; implications for comorbidity. *Journal of Nervous and Mental Disease*, **183**, 304–308.

Bandura, A. (1969). Modelling approaches to the modification of phobic disorders. *International Psychiatry Clinics*, **6**, 201–223.

Barlow, D.H. (1985). The dimensions of anxiety disorders. In: *Anxiety and the Anxiety Disorders* (eds. Tuma, A.H., & Maser, J.D.), pp. 479–500. Hillsdale, New Jersey: Lawrence Erlbaum.

Barlow, D.H. (1987). The classification of anxiety. In: *Diagnosis and Classification of Psychiatry: A Critical Appraisal of DSM-III* (ed. Tischler, G.), pp. 221–242. Cambridge: Cambridge University Press.

Barlow, D.H. (1988). *Anxiety and Its Disorders: The Nature and Treatment of Anxiety and Panic.* New York: Guilford Press.

Barlow, D.H., Cohen, A.S., Waddell, M., Vermilyea, J.A., Klosko, J.S., Blanchard, E.B., & DiNardo, P.A. (1984). Panic and generalized anxiety disorders: nature and treatment. *Behavior Therapy*, **15**, 431–439.

Barlow, D.H., DiNardo, P.A., Vermilyea, B.B., Vermilyea, J.A., & Blanchard, E.B. (1986). Co-morbidity and depression among the anxiety disorders: issues in diagnosis and classification. *Journal of Nervous and Mental Disease*, **174**, 63–72.

Barsky, A.J., & Klerman, G.L. (1983). Overview: hypochondriasis, bodily complaints, and somatic styles. *American Journal of Psychiatry*, **140**, 273–283.

Barsky, A.J., Wyshak, G., & Klerman, G.L. (1992). Psychiatric comorbidity in DSM-III-R hypochondriasis. *Archives of General Psychiatry*, **49**, 101–108.

Barsky, A.J., Barnett, M.C., & Cleary, P.D. (1994). Hypochondriasis and panic disorder: boundary and overlap. *Archives of General Psychiatry*, **51**, 918–925.

Basoglu, M., Marks, I.M., Kilic, C., Brewin, C.R., & Swinson, R.P. (1994). Alprazolam and exposure for panic disorder with agoraphobia: attribution of improvement predicts subsequent relapse. *British Journal of Psychiatry*, **164**, 652–659.

Battaglia, M., Bernardeschi, L., Politi, E., Bertella, S., & Bellodi, L. (1995). Comorbidity of panic and somatization disorder: a genetic-epidemiological approach. *Comprehensive Psychiatry*, **36**, 411–420.

Beck, A.T. (1976). *Cognitive Therapy and the Emotional Disorders.* New York: International Universities Press.

Beck, A.T., Emery, G., & Greenberg, R.L. (1985). *Anxiety Disorders and Phobias: A Cognitive Perspective.* New York: Basic Books.

Birkett, P., & Tyrer, P. (1990). Beta-blocking drugs for the treatment of anxiety disorder. In: *Handbook of Anxiety – Volume 4.* (eds. Noyes, R. Jr., Roth, M., & Burrows, G.D.), pp. 147–168. Amsterdam: Elsevier.

Blanchard, E.B., Appelbaum, K.A., Nicholson, N.L., Radnitz, C.L., Morrill, B., Michultka, D., Kirsch, C., Hillhouse, J., & Dentinger, M.P. (1990). A controlled evaluation of the addition of cognitive therapy to a home-based biofeedback and relaxation treatment of vascular headache. *Headache.* **30**, 371–376.

Bond, A.J., & Lader, M.H. (1974). The use of analog scales in rating subjective feelings. *British Journal of Medical Psychology,* **47**, 211–218.

Bonn, J.A., Turner, P., & Hicks, D.C. (1972). Beta-adrenergic-receptor blockade with practolol in treatment of anxiety. *The Lancet,* **1**, 814–815.

Boulenger, J.P. (1995). Le traitement de l'anxiété generalisée: approches pharmacologiques nouvelles. *l'Encephale,* **21**, 459–466.

Bowlby, J. (1973). *Attachment and Loss – Volume 2, Separation: Anxiety and Anger.* London: Hogarth Press.

Boyd, J.H., Burke, J.D., Gruenberg, E., Holzer, C.E., Rae, D.S., George, L.K., Karno, M., Svoltzman, R., McEvoy, L., & Nestadt, G. (1984). Exclusion criteria of DSM-III: a study of co-occurrence of hierarchy-free syndromes. *Archives of General Psychiatry,* **41**, 983–989.

Braun, D.L., Sunday, S.R., & Halmi, K.A. (1994). Psychiatric comorbidity in patients with eating disorders. *Psychological Medicine,* **24**, 859–867.

Brawman-Mintzer, O., Lydiard, R.B., Emmanuel, N., Payeur, R., Johnson, M., Roberts, J., Jarrell, M.P., & Ballenger, J.C. (1993). Psychiatric comorbidity in patients with generalized anxiety disorder. *American Journal of Psychiatry,* **150**, 1216–1218.

Breier, A., Charney, D.S., & Heninger, G.R. (1984). Major depression in patients with agoraphobia and panic disorder. *Archives of General Psychiatry,* **41**, 1129–1135.

Brewin, C.R. (1996). Theoretical foundations of cognitive-behavior therapy for anxiety and depression. *Annual Review of Psychology,* **47**, 33–57.

Briggs, A.C., Stretch, D.D., & Brandon, S. (1993). Subtyping of panic disorder by symptom profile. *British Journal of Psychiatry,* **163**, 201–209.

Bronisch, T., & Wittchen, H.U. (1994). Suicidal ideation and suicide attempts: comorbidity with depression, anxiety disorders, and substance abuse disorder. *European Archives of Psychiatry and Clinical Neuroscience*, **244**, 93–98.

Bronisch, T., & Hecht, H. (1990). Major depression with and without a coexisting anxiety disorder: social dysfunction, social integration, and personality features. *Journal of Affective Disorders*, **20**, 151–157.

Brown, C., & Schulberg, H.C. (1995). The efficacy of psychosocial treatments in primary care: a review of randomised clinical trials. *General Hospital Psychiatry*, **17**, 414–424.

Brown, F.W., Golding, J.M., & Smith, G.R.J. (1990). Psychiatric comorbidity in primary care somatization disorder. *Psychosomatic Medicine*, **52**, 445–451.

Brown, G.W., & Harris, T.O. (1978). Social origins of depression. London: Tavistock Press.

Brown, G.W., & Harris, T.O. (1993). Aetiology of anxiety and depressive disorders in an inner-city population. 1. Early adversity. *Psychological Medicine*, **23**, 143–154.

Brown, G.W., Harris, T.O., & Eales, M.J. (1993). Aetiology of anxiety and depressive disorders in an inner-city population. 2. Comorbidity and adversity. *Psychological Medicine*, **23**, 155–165.

Brown, G.W., Lemyre, L., & Bifulco, A. (1992). Social factors and recovery from anxiety and depressive disorders: a test of specificity. *British Journal of Psychiatry*, **161**, 44–54.

Brown, T.A., & Barlow, D.H. (1992). Comorbidity among anxiety disorders: implications for treatment and DSM-IV. *Journal of Consulting and Clinical Psychology*, **60**, 835–844.

Brown, T.A., & Barlow, D.H. (1995). Long-term outcome in cognitive-behavioral treatment of panic disorder: clinical predictors and alternative strategies for assessment. *Journal of Consulting and Clinical Psychology*, **63**, 754–765.

Brown, T.A., Antony, M.A., & Barlow, D.H. (1995). Diagnostic comorbidity in panic disorder: effect on treatment outcome and course of comorbid diagnoses following treatment. *Journal of Consulting and Clinical Psychology*, **63**, 404–418.

Butler, G. (1993). Predicting outcome after treatment for generalised anxiety disorder. *Behaviour Research and Therapy*, **31**, 211–213.

Butler, G., Cullington, A., Hibbert, G., Klines, I., & Gelder, M. (1987). Anxiety management for persistent generalised anxiety. *British Journal of Psychiatry*, **151**, 535–542.

Butler, G., Fennell, M., Robson, P., & Gelder, M. (1991). Comparison of behavior therapy and cognitive behavior therapy in the treatment of generalized anxiety disorder. *Journal of Consulting and Clinical Psychology*, **59**, 167–175.

Canter, A., Condo, C.Y., & Knott, J.R. (1975). A comparison of EMG feedback and progressive muscular relaxation in anxiety neurosis. *British Journal of Psychiatry*, **127**, 470–475.

Cassidy, S.L., & Henry, J.A. (1987). Fatal toxicity of antidepressant drugs in overdose. *British Medical Journal*, **295**, 1021–1024.

Castillo, C.S., Schultz, S.K., & Robinson, R.G. (1995). Clinical correlates of early-onset and late-onset poststroke generalized anxiety. *American Journal of Psychiatry*, **152**, 1174–1179.

Cattell, R.B. (1957). *Handbook for I.P.A.T. Anxiety Scale*. Champaign, Illinois: Institute for Personality and Ability Testing.

Chambless, D. (1985). The relationship of severity of agoraphobia to associated psychopathology. *Behaviour Research and Therapy*, **23**, 305–310.

Charney, D.S., & Deutch, A. (1996). A functional neuroanatomy of anxiety and fear: implications for the pathophysiology and treatment of anxiety disorders. *Critical Reviews in Neurobiology*, **10**, 419–446.

Charney, D.S., & Redmond, D.E., Jr. (1983). Neurobiological mechanisms in human anxiety. Evidence supporting central noradrenergic hyperactivity. *Neuropharmacology*, **22**, 1531–1536.

Charney, D.S., Heninger, G.R., & Jatlow, P.I. (1985). Increased anxiogenic effects of caffeine in panic disorders. *Archives of General Psychiatry*, **42**, 233–243.

Charney, D.S., Woods, S.W., Goodman, W.K., & Heninger, G.R. (1987). Neurobiological mechanisms of panic anxiety: biochemical and behavioral correlates of yohimbine-induced panic attacks. *American Journal of Psychiatry*, **144**, 1030–1036.

Clark, D.M. (1986). A cognitive approach to panic. *Behaviour, Research and Therapy*, **24**, 461–470.

Clark, D.M. (1990). Cognitive therapy for depression and anxiety: is it better than drug treatment in the long term. In: *Dilemmas and Difficulties in the Management of Psychiatric Patients* (eds. Hawton, K., & Cowen, P.), pp. 55–64. Oxford: Oxford University Press.

Cloninger, C.R. (1987). *Tridimensional Personality Questionnaire (TPQ)*. Department of Psychiatry and Genetics, Washington University School of Medicine, St Louis, Missouri.

Committee on Review of Medicines (1980). Systematic review of the benzodiazepines. *British Medical Journal,* 2, 719–720.

Cottraux, J., Note, I.D., Cungi, C., Legeron, P., Heim, F., Chneiweiss, L., Bernard, G., & Bouvard, M. (1995). A controlled study of cognitive behaviour therapy with buspirone or placebo in panic disorder with agoraphobia. *British Journal of Psychiatry,* 167, 635–641.

Cowen, P.J., & Nutt, D.J. (1982). Abstinence symptoms after withdrawal of tranqillising drugs: is there a common neurochemical mechanism? *The Lancet,* 1, 360–362.

Daly, R.J. (1983). Samuel Pepys and post traumatic stress disorder. *British Journal of Psychiatry,* 143, 64–68.

Darwin, C. (1872). *Emotional and Expression in Man and Other Animals.* London: Longmans.

Dawson, G.D. (1951). A summation technique for detecting small signals in a large irregular background. *Journal of Physiology,* 115, 2P–3P.

Delini-Stula, A., Mikkelsen, H., & Angst, J. (1995). Therapeutic efficacy of antidepressants in agitated anxious depression — A meta-analysis of moclobemide studies. *Journal of Affective Disorders,* 35, 21–30.

Deltito, J.A., & Stam, M. (1989). Psychopharmacological treatment of avoidant personality disorder. *Comprehensive Psychiatry,* 30, 498–504.

Den Boer, J.A., Westenberg, H.G.M., & Kamerbeek, W.D.J. (1987). Effect of serotonin uptake inhibitors in anxiety disorders: a double-blind comparison of clomipramine and fluvoxamine. *International Clinical Psychopharmacology,* 2, 21–32.

Derogatis, L.R., Lipman, R.S., & Covi, L. (1974). The SCL-90: an outpatient psychiatric rating scale. *Psychopharmacology Bulletin,* 9, 13–28.

Dilsaver, S.C. (1994). Withdrawal phenomena associated with antidepressant and antipsychotic agents. *Drug Safety*, **10**, 103–114.

Dixon, N.F. (1971) *Subliminal Perception: The Nature of a Controversy*. London: McGraw-Hill.

Donnan, P., Hutchinson, A., & Paxton, R. (1990). Self help materials for anxiety: a randomised controlled trial in general practice. *British Journal of General Practice*, **40**, 498–501.

Dreessen, L., Arntz, A., Luttels, C., & Sallaerts, S. (1994). Personality disorders do not influence the results of cognitive behavior therapies for anxiety disorders. *Comprehensive Psychiatry*, **35**, 265–274.

Drugs and Therapeutics Bulletin. (1993). Psychological treatment for anxiety — An alternative to drugs? *Drug and Therapeutics Bulletin*, **31**, 73–75.

Dunbar, G.C., Cohn, J.B., Fabre, L.F., Feighner, J.P., Fieve, R.R., Mendels, J., & Shrivastava, R.K. (1991). A comparison of paroxetine, imipramine and placebo in depressed out-patients. *British Journal of Psychiatry*, **159**, 394–398.

Durham, R.C., & Allan, T. (1993). Psychological treatment of generalised anxiety disorder. A review of the clinical significance of results in outcome studies since 1980. *British Journal of Psychiatry*, **163**, 19–26.

Durham, R.C., Murphy, T., Allan, T., Richard, K., Treliving, L.R., & Fenton, G.W. (1994). Cognitive therapy, analytic psychotherapy and anxiety management training for generalised anxiety disorder. *British Journal of Psychiatry*, **165**, 315–323.

Eison, M.S. (1990). Serotonin: a common neurobiologic substrate in anxiety and depression. *Journal of Clinical Psychopharmacology (Suppl 3)*, **10**, 26–30.

Eliasch, H., Lager, C.G., Norrback, K., Rosen, A., & Scott, H. (1967). The beta-adrenergic receptor blockade modification of the systematic haemodynamic effects of link trainer simulated flight. *Forsvarmedecin*, 120–129.

Elkin, I., Shea, M.T., Watkins, J.T., Imber, S.D., Sotsky, S.M., Collins, J.F., Glass, D.R., Pilkonis, P.A., Leber, W.R., Docherty, J.P., *et al.* (1989). National Institute of Mental Health Treatment of

Depression Collaborative Research Program. General effectiveness of treatments. *Archives of General Psychiatry*, **46**, 971–982.

Emmanuel, J.S., Simmonds, S., & Tyrer, P. (1998). A systematic review of the outcome of anxiety and depressive disorders. *British Journal of Psychiatry (Suppl 34)*, **173**, 35–41.

Emmelkamp, P.M.G., & Kuipers, A.C.M. (1979). Agoraphobia: a follow-up study 4 years after treatment. *British Journal of Psychiatry*, **134**, 352–355.

Faravelli, C., & Albanesi, G. (1987). Agoraphobia with panic attacks: one-year prospective follow-up. *Comprehensive Psychiatry*, **28**, 481–487.

Farmer, R.D.T., & Pinder, R.M. (1989). Why do fatal overdose rates vary between antidepressants? *Acta Psychiatrica Scandinavica (Suppl 354)*, **80**, 25–35.

Feighner, J.P., Merideth, C.H., & Hendrickson, G.A. (1982). A double-blind comparison of buspirone and diazepam in out-patients with generalised anxiety disorder. *Journal of Clinical Psychiatry — Section 2*, **43**, 103–107.

Feinstein, A. (1970). The pre-therapeutic classification of comorbidity in chronic disease. *Journal of Chronic Diseases*, **23**, 455–462.

Ferguson, J.M., Taylor, C.B., & Wermuth, B. (1978). Rapid behavioral treatment for needle phobics. *Journal of Nervous and Mental Disease*, **166**, 294–298.

Fink, P. (1995). Psychiatric illness in patients with persistent somatisation. *British Journal of Psychiatry*, **166**, 93–99.

Flick, S.N., Roy-Byrne, P.P., Cowley, D.S., Shores, M.M., & Dunner, D.L. (1993). DSM-III-R personality disorders in a mood and anxiety disorders clinic: prevalence, comorbidity and clinical correlates. *Journal of Affective Disorders*, **27**, 71–79.

Foa, E.B., Rothbaum, B.O., Riggs, D.S., & Murdock, T.B. (1991). Treatment of posttraumatic stress disorder in rape victims: a comparison between cognitive-behavioral procedures and counseling. *Journal of Consulting and Clinical Psychology*, **59**, 715–723.

Fontaine, R., Chouinard, G., & Annable, L. (1984). Rebound anxiety in anxious patients after abrupt withdrawal of benzodiazepine treatment. *American Journal of Psychiatry*, **141**, 848–852.

Fontaine, R., Beaudry, P., Beauclair, L., & Chouinard, G. (1987). Comparison of withdrawal of buspirone and diazepam: a placebo controlled trial. *Progress in Neuropsychology and Biological Psychiatry*, **11**, 189–197.

Freud, S. (1895). On the grounds for detaching a particular syndrome from newurasthenia inder the description "anxiety neurosis". In: *Complete Psychological Works — Volume 3*. (ed. Strachey, J.T.), pp. 85–117. London: Hogarth Press.

Freud, S. (1908). Character and anal-eroticism. In: *Complete Psychological Works* (ed. Strachey, J.T.), pp. 167–175. London: Hogarth Press.

Freud, S. (1926). Inhibitions, symptoms and anxiety. In: *Complete Psychological Works — Volume 20*. (ed. Strachey, J.T.), pp. 75–174. London: Hogarth Press.

Fromm, E. (1942). *Fear of Freedom*. London: Routledge.

Geddes, J.R., & Harrison, P.J. (1997). Closing the gap between research and practice. *British Journal of Psychiatry*, **171**, 220–225.

Gelder, M.G. (1986). Panic attacks: new approaches to an old problem. *British Journal of Psychiatry*, **149**, 346–352.

George, D.T., Nutt, D.J., Dwyer, B.A., & Linnoila, M. (1990). Alcoholism and panic disorder: is the comorbidity more than coincidence? *Acta Psychiatrica Scandinavica*, **81**, 97–107.

Ghosh, A., & Marks, I.M. (1987). Self-treatment of agoraphobia by exposure. *Behavior Therapy*, **18**, 3–16.

Gilberstadt, H., & Maley, M. (1965). GSR, clinical state and psychiatric diagnosis. *Journal of Clinical Psychology*, **21**, 233–238.

Goldberg, D., Bridges, K., Duncan-Jones, P., & Grayson, D. (1987). Dimensions of neuroses seen in primary care settings. *Psychological Medicine*, **17**, 461–471.

Goldberg, D., Bridges, K., Cook, D., Evans, B., & Grayson, D. (1990). The influence of social factors on common mental disorders: destabilisation and restitution. *British Journal of Psychiatry*, **156**, 704–713.

Goldberg, D., & Huxley, P. (1992). *Common Mental Disorders: A Biosocial Model*. London: Tavistock Routledge.

Goodman, W.K., Price, L.H., Rasmussen, S.A., Mazure, C., Delgado, P., Heninger, G.R., & Charney, D.S. (1989). The Yale-Brown Obsessive Compulsive Scale. II. Validity. *Archives of General Psychiatry*, **46**, 1012–1016.

Granville-Grossman, K.L., & Turner, P. (1966). The effect of propranolol on anxiety. *Lancet*, **i**, 788–790.

Gray, J.A. (1976). The behavioural inhibition system: a possible substrate for anxiety. In: *Theoretical and Experimental Bases of Behaviour Modification* (eds. Feldman, M.P., & Broadhurst, A.M.), pp. 3–41. Chichester: John Wiley.

Gray, J.A. (1982). *The Neuropsychology of Anxiety: An Enquiry into the Functions of the Septo-Hippocampal System.* Oxford: Clarendon Press.

Greenblatt, D.J., & Shader, R. I. (1974). *Benzodiazepines in Clinical Practice.* New York: Raven Press.

Greene, B., & Blanchard, E.B. (1994). Cognitive therapy for irritable bowel syndrome. *Journal of Consulting and Clinical Psychology*, **62**, 576–582.

Greer, H.S., & Cawley, R.H. (1966). Some observations on the natural history of neurotic illness. In: Anonymous, *Australian Medical Association, Mervyn Archdall Medical Monograph — Number 3.* Glebe, Australia: Australasian Medical Publishing Company.

Griffiths, R.R., & Weerts, E.M. (1997). Benzodiazepine self-administration in humans and laboratory animals: implications for problems of long-term use and abuse, *Psychopharmacology*, **134**, 1–37.

Guze, S.B. (1967). The diagnosis of hysteria: what are we trying to do? *American Journal of Psychiatry*, **123**, 491–498.

Guze, S.B., Woodruff, R.A., & Clayton, P.J. (1971). Hysteria and antisocial personality: further evidence of an association. *American Journal of Psychiatry*, **127**, 957–960.

Guze, S.B., Cloninger, C.R., Martin, R.L., & Clayton, P.J. (1986). A follow-up and family study of Briquet's syndrome. *British Journal of Psychiatry*, **149**, 17–23.

Haddad, P. (1997). Newer antidepressants and the discontinuation syndrome. *Journal of Clinical Psychiatry (Suppl 7)*, **58**, 17–21.

Hallam, R.S. (1978). Agoraphobia: a critical review of the concept. *British Journal of Psychiatry*, **133**, 314–319.

Hamilton, M. (1959). The assessment of anxiety states by rating. *British Journal of Medical Psychology*, **32**, 50–55.

Haver, B., & Dahlgren, L. (1995). Early treatment of women with alcohol addiction (EWA): a comprehensive evaluation and outcome study. I. Patterns of psychiatric comorbidity at intake. *Addiction*, **90**, 101–109.

Hecht, H., von Zerssen, D., & Wittchen, H.U. (1990). Anxiety and depression in a community sample: the influence of comorbidity on social functioning. *Journal of Affective Disorders*, **18**, 137–144.

Hecht, H., von Zerssen, D., Krieg, C., Possl, J., & Wittchen, H.U. (1989). Anxiety and depression: comorbidity, psychopathology, and social functioning. *Comprehensive Psychiatry*, **30**, 420–433.

Hecker, E. (1893). Über larvirte und abortive Angstzustände bei Neurasthenie. *Zentralblatt für Nervenheilkunde und Psychiatrie (Berlin)*, **133**, 565–572.

Heimberg, R.G., & Barlow, D. H. (1991). New developments in cognitive-behavioral therapy for social phobia. *Journal of Clinical Psychiatry*, (*Suppl*), **52**, 21–30.

Helzer, J.E., & Pryzbeck, T.R. (1988). The co-occurrence of alcoholism with other psychiatric disorders in the general population and its impact on treatment. *Journal of Studies on Alcohol*, **49**, 219–224.

Herbert, J.D., Hope, D.A., & Bellack, A.S. (1992). Validity of the distinction between generalized social phobia and avoidant personality disorder. *Journal of Abnormal Psychology*, **101**, 332–339.

Hodes, M. (1993). Anorexia nervosa and bulimia nervosa in children. *International Review of Psychiatry*, **5**, 101–108.

Hoehn-Saric, R. (1981). Characteristics of chronic anxiety patients. In: *Anxiety: New Research and Changing Concepts* (eds. Klein, D.F., & Rabkin, J.G.), pp. 399–409. New York: Raven Press.

Hoehn-Saric, R. (1982). Comparison of generalized anxiety disorder with panic disorder patients. *Psychopharmacological Bulletin*, **18**, 104–109.

Hoehn-Saric, R., & McLeod, D.R. (1985). Generalized anxiety disorder. *Psychiatric Clinics of North America*, **8**, 73–88.

Hoffart, A., Thornes, K., & Hedley, L.M. (1995). DSM-III-R Axis I and II disorders in agoraphobic inpatients with and without panic disorder before and after psychosocial treatment. *Psychiatry Research*, **56**, 1–9.

Holton, A., & Tyrer, P. (1990). Five year outcome of patients withdrawn from long-term treatment with diazepam. *British Medical Journal*, **300**, 1241–1242.

Holton, A., Riley, P., & Tyrer, P. (1992). Factors predicting long-term outcome after chronic benzodiazepine therapy. *Journal of Affective Disorders*, **24**, 245–252.

Hudson, J.I., & Pope, H.G.J. (1990). Affective spectrum disorder: does antidepressant response identify a family of disorders with a common pathophysiology? *American Journal of Psychiatry*, **147**, 552–564.

Huxley, P.J., Goldberg, D., Maguire, P., & Kincey, V. (1979). The prediction of the course of minor psychiatric disorders. *British Journal of Psychiatry*, **135**, 535–543.

Imber, S.D., Pilkonis, P.A., Sotsky, S.M., Elkin, I., Watkins, J.T., Collins, J.F., Shea, M.T., Leber, W.R., & Glass, D.R. (1990). Mode-specific effects among three treatments for depression. *Journal of Consulting and Clinical Psychology*, **58**, 352–359.

Insel, T., & Johar, J. (1987). Psychopharmacologic approaches to obsessive-compulsive disorder. In: *Psychopharmacology: The Third Generation of Progress* (ed. Meltzer, H.Y.), pp. 1205–1210. New York: Raven Press.

Jacobson, E. (1939). *Progressive Relaxation*. Chicago: University of Chicago Press.

James, I.M., Pearson, R.M., Griffith, D.N.W., & Newbury, P. (1977). The effect of oxprenolol on stage fright in musicians. *The Lancet*, **2**, 952.

James, I.M., & Temple-Savage, I. (1984). Beneficial effects of nadolol on anxiety induced disturbance of performance in musicians: a comparison with diazepam and placebo. *American Heart Journal*, **108**, 1150–1155.

James, I.M., Burgoyne, W., & Savage, I.T. (1983). Effect of pindolol on stress-related disturbances of musical performances: preliminary communication. *Journal of the Royal Society of Medicine*, **76**, 194–196.

James, W. (1891). *Principles of Psychology*. London: Longman.

Jardine, R., Martin, N.G., & Henderson, A.S. (1984). Genetic covariation between neuroticism and the symptoms of anxiety and depression. *Genetic Epidemiology*, 1, 89–107.

Johnson, J., Weissman, M.M., & Klerman, G.L. (1990). Panic disorder, comorbidity, and suicide attempts. *Archives of General Psychiatry*, 47, 805–808.

Johnstone, E.C., Cunningham Owens, D.G., Frith, C.D., McPherson, K., & Dowie, C. (1980). Neurotic illness and its response to anxiolytic and anti-depressant treatment. *Psychological Medicine*, 10, 321–328.

Kagan, J., Kearsley, R., & Zelaso, P. (1978). *Infancy: Its Place in Human Development*. Cambridge, Massachusetts: Harvard University Press.

Kahn, R.J., McNair, D.M., Lipman, R.S., Covi, L., Rickels, K., Downing, R.W., Fisher, S., & Frankenthaler, L.M. (1986). Imipramine and chlordiazepoxide in depressive and anxiety disorders: II. Efficacy in anxious out-patients. *Archives of General Psychiatry*, 43, 79–85.

Kardiner, A. (1941). *The Traumatic Neuroses of War*. New York: Hoeber.

Kasper, S., Moller, H.J., Montgomery, S.A., & Zondag, E. (1995). Antidepressant efficacy in relation to item analysis and severity of depression: a placebo-controlled trial of fluvoxamine versus imipramine. *International Clinical Psychopharmacology* (*Suppl 4*), 9, 3–12.

Katon, W., Hollifield, M., Chapman, T., Mannuzza, S., Ballenger, J., & Fyer, A. (1995). Infrequent panic attacks: psychiatric comorbidity, personality characteristics and functional disability. *Journal of Psychiatric Research*, 29, 121–131.

Kelly, D.H.W., & Walter, C.J.S. (1968). The relationship between clinical diagnosis and anxiety, assessed by forearm blood flow and other measurements. *British Journal of Psychiatry*, 114, 611–626.

Kendell, R.E. (1974). The stability of psychiatric diagnoses. *British Journal of Psychiatry*, 124, 352–356.

Kendell, R.E. (1989). Clinical validity. *Psychological Medicine*, 19, 45–55.

Kendler, K.S., Neale, M.C., Kessler, R.C., Heath, A.C., & Eaves, L.J. (1992). Major depression and generalized anxiety disorder. Same genes (partly) different environments? *Archives of General Psychiatry*, **49**, 716–722.

Kendler, K.S., Walters, E.E., Neale, M.C., Kessler, R.C., Heath, A.C., & Eaves, L.J. (1995). The structure of the genetic and environmental risk factors for six major psychiatric disorders in women. Phobia, generalized anxiety disorder, panic disorder, bulimia, major depression, and alcoholism. *Archives of General Psychiatry*, **52**, 374–383.

Kenyon, F.E. (1965). Hypochondriasis: a survey of some historical, clinical and social aspects. *British Journal of Medical Psychology*, **38**, 117–133.

Kerr, T.A., Roth, M., & Schapira, K. (1974). Prediction of outcome in anxiety states and depressive illnesses. *British Journal of Psychiatry*, **124**, 125–133.

Kerr, T.A., Roth, M., Schapira, K., & Gurney, C. (1972). The assessment and prediction of outcome in affective disorders. *British Journal of Psychiatry*, **121**, 167–174.

Kessler, R.C., McGonagle, K.A., Zhao, S., Nelson, C.B., Hughes, M., Eshleman, S., Wittchen, H.U., & Kendler, K.S. (1994). Lifetime and 12-month prevalence of DSM-III-R psychiatric disorders in the United States. Results from the National Comorbidity Survey. *Archives of General Psychiatry*, **51**, 8–19.

Kessler, R.C., Nelson, C.B., McGonagle, K.A., Edlund, M.J., Frank, R.G., & Leaf, P.J. (1996). The epidemiology of co-occurring addictive and mental disorders; implications for prevention and service utilization. *American Journal of Orthopsychiatry*, **66**, 17–31.

Kingdon, D., Tyrer, P., Seivewright, N., Ferguson, B., & Murphy, S. (1996). The Nottingham Study of Neurotic Disorder: influence of cognitive therapists on outcome. *British Journal of Psychiatry*, **169**, 93–97.

Klein, D.F. (1964). Delineation of two drug-responsive anxiety syndromes. *Psychopharmacologia*, **5**, 397–408.

Klein, D.F. (1967). Importance of psychiatric diagnosis in prediction of clinical drug effects. *Archives of General Psychiatry*, **16**, 118–125.

Klein, D.F. (1980). Anxiety reconceptualized. *Comprehensive Psychiatry*, **21**, 411–427.

Klein, D.F. (1981). Anxiety reconceptualized. In: *Anxiety, New Research and Changing Concepts* (eds. Klein, D.F., & Rabkin, J.G.), pp. 235–263. New York: Raven Press.

Klerman, G.L. (1988). Principles of interpersonal psychotherapy for depression. In: *Depression and Mania* (eds. Georgotas, A. & Cancro, R.), pp. 490–501. Amsterdam: Elsevier.

Lacey, J.I., Bateman, D.E., & Vanlehn, R. (1953). Autonomic response specificity: an experimental study. *Psychosomatic Medicine,* 15, 8–21.

Lader, M. (1988). The practical use of buspirone. In Buspirone: a new introduction to the treatment of anxiety. *Journal of the Royal Society of Medicine,* 71–76.

Lader, M., Beaumont, G., Bond, A., Butler, G., Cobb, J., Ghosh, A., Hallstrom, C., Ritchie, L., & Tyrer, P. (1992). Guidelines for the management of patients with generalised anxiety. *Psychiatric Bulletin,* 16, 560–565.

Lader, M.H., & Wing, L. (1966). *Physiological Measures, Sedative Drugs and Morbid Anxiety.* London: Oxford University Press.

Lader, M.H. (1967). Palmar skin conductance measures in anxiety and phobic states. *Journal of Psychosomatic Research,* 11, 271–281.

Larkin, B.A., Copeland, J.R.M., Dewey, M.E., Davidson, I.A., Saunders, P.A., Sharma, V.K., McWilliam, C., & Sullivan, C. (1992). The natural history of neurotic disorder in an elderly urban population: findings from the Liverpool study of continuing health in the community. *British Journal of Psychiatry,* 160, 681–686.

Lazare, A., Klerman, G.L., & Armor, D.J. (1966). Oral, obsessive and hysterical personality patterns. *Archives of General Psychiatry,* 14, 624–630.

Lee, I., & Tyrer, P. (1981). Self-report and physiological responses to subliminal and supraliminal motion pictures. *Journal of Nervous and Mental Disease,* 169, 165–169.

Lee, I., Tyrer, P., & Horn, S. (1983). A comparison of subliminal, supraliminal and faded phobic cine-films in the treatment of agoraphobia. *British Journal of Psychiatry,* 143, 356–361.

Lelliott, P.T., Marks, I.M., Monteiro, W.O., Tsakiris, F., & Noshirvani, H. (1987). Agoraphobics 5 years after imipramine and exposure.

Outcome and predictors. *Journal of Nervous and Mental Disease*, **175**, 599–605.

Lepola, U. (1994). Alcohol and depression in panic disorder. *Acta Psychiatrica Scandinavica (Suppl)*, **377**, 33–35.

Lesser, I.M., Rubin, R.T., Pecknold, J.C., Rifkin, A., Swinson, R.P., Lydiard, R.B., Burrows, G.D., Noyes, R.J., & DuPont, R.L.J. (1988). Secondary depression in panic disorder and agoraphobia. I. Frequency, severity, and response to treatment. *Archives of General Psychiatry*, **45**, 437–443.

Lewis A. (1967). Problems presented by the ambiguous word "anxiety" as used in psychopathology. *Israel Annals of Psychiatry and Related Disciplines*, **5**, 105–121.

Lewis, A.J. (1934). Melancholia: a historical review. *Journal of Mental Science*, **80**, 1–42.

Lidren, D.M., Watkins, P.L., Gould, R.A., Clum, G.A., Asterino, M., & Tulloch, H.L. (1994). A comparison of bibliotherapy and group therapy in the treatment of panic disorder. *Journal of Consulting and Clinical Psychology*, **62**, 865–869.

Lipman, R.S., Covi, L., Rickels, K., McNair, D.M., Downing, R., Kahn, R.J., Lasseter, V.K., & Faden, V. (1986). Imipramine and chlordiazepoxide in depressive and anxiety disorders: I. Efficacy in depressed out-patients. *Archives of General Psychiatry*, **43**, 68–77.

Lipowski, Z.J. (1988). Somatization: the concept and its clinical application. *American Journal of Psychiatry*, **145**, 1358–1368.

Loranger, A.W., Sartorius, N., Andreoli, A., Berger, P., Buchheim, P., Channabasavanna, S.M., Coid, B., Dahl, A., Diekstra, R.F., Ferguson, B., *et al.* (1994). The International Personality Disorder Examination. The World Health Organization/Alcohol, Drug Abuse, and Mental Health Administration international pilot study of personality disorders.*Archives of General Psychiatry*, **51**, 215–224.

Lyons, M.J., Tyrer, P., Gunderson, J., & Tohen, M. (1997). Heuristic models of comorbidity of axis I and axis II disorders. *Journal of Personality Disorders*, **11**, 260–269.

Macalpine, I., & Hunter, R. (1969). *George III and the Mad Business.* London: Allen Lane.

McLean, P.D. (1955). The limbic system (visceral brain) and emotional behaviour. *Archives of Neurology and Psychiatry,* **73**, 130–134.

Mannuzza, S., Schneier, F.R., Chapman, T.F., Liebowitz, M.R., Klein, D.F., & Fyer, A.J. (1995). Generalized social phobia. Reliability and validity. *Archives of General Psychiatry,* **52**, 230–237.

Margraf, J., Taylor, C.B., Ehlers, A., Roth, W.T., & Agras, W.S. (1987). Panic attacks in the natural environment. *Journal of Nervous and Mental Disease,* **175**, 558–565.

Marks, I.M. (1970). The classification of phobic disorders. *British Journal of Psychiatry,* **116**, 377–386.

Marks, I.M. (1987). *Fears, Phobias and Rituals.* Oxford: Oxford University Press.

Marks, I., & Marks, M. (1990). Exposure treatment of agoraphobia/panic. In: *Handbook of Anxiety — Volume 4, The Treatment of Anxiety* (eds. Noyes, R. Jr., Roth, M., & Burrows, G.D.), pp. 293–310. Amsterdam: Elsevier.

Marks, I.M., Gelder, M.G., & Edwards, G. (1966). Hypnosis and desensitisation for phobias: a controlled clinical trial. *British Journal of Psychiatry,* **114**, 1263–1268.

Marks, I.M., & Mathews, A.M. (1979). Standard self-rating for phobic patients. *Behaviour Research and Therapy,* **17**, 263–267.

Mathews, A.M., Gelder, M.G., & Johnston, D.W. (1981). *Agoraphobia: Nature and Treatment.* Oxford: Oxford University Press.

McGuffin, P., Farmer, A.E., & Harvey, I. (1991). A polydiagnostic application of operational criteria in studies of psychotic illness: development and reliability of the OPCRIT system. *Archives of General Psychiatry,* **48**, 764–770.

Mellman, T.A., & Uhde, T.W. (1987). Obsessive-compulsive symptoms in panic disorder. *American Journal of Psychiatry,* **144**, 1573–1576.

Meltzer, H., Gill, B., & Petticrew, M. (1994). *OPCS Surveys of Psychiatric Morbidity in Great Britain. Bulletin Number 1: The Prevalence of Psychiatric Morbidity Among Adults Aged 16–64 — Living in Private Households, in Great Britain.* London: OPCS.

Merikangas, K.R., & Angst, J. (1995). Comorbidity and social phobia: evidence from clinical, epidemiologic, and genetic studies. *European Archiver of Psychiatry and Clinical Neuroscience*, **244**, 297–303.

Mischel, W. (1973). Towards a cognitive social learning reconceptualization of personality. *Psychological Review*, **80**, 252–283.

Montgomery, S.A. (1993). Obsessive compulsive disorder is not an anxiety disorder. *International Clinical Psychopharmacology (Suppl 1)*, **8**, 57–62.

Montgomery, S.A., & Åsberg, M. (1979). A new depression scale designed to be sensitive to change. *British Journal of Psychiatry*, **134**, 382–389.

Montgomery, S.A., Montgomery, D.B., Green, M., Bullock, T., & Baldwin, D. (1992). Pharmacotherapy in the prevention of suicidal behavior. *Journal of Clinical Psychopharmacology*, **12**, 27S–31S.

Monti, J.M., Attali, P., Monti, D., Zipfel, A., de la Giclais, B., & Morselli, P.L. (1994). Zolpidem and rebound insomnia — A double-blind, controlled polysomnographic study in chronic insomniac patients. *Pharmacopsychiatry*, **27**, 166–175.

Mott, F.W. (1918). Two addresses on war psychoneuroses. *Lancet*, **i**, 127–129 and 169–172.

Munro, A. (1966). Some familial and social factors in depressive illness. *British Journal of Psychiatry*, **112**, 429–437.

Murphy, J.M., Olivier, D.C., Sobol, A.M., Monson, R.R., & Leighton, A.H. (1986). Diagnosis and outcome: depression and anxiety in a general population. *Psychological Medicine*, **16**, 117–126.

Murphy, S.M., & Tyrer, P. (1991). A double-blind comparison of the effects of gradual withdrawal of lorazepam, diazepam and bromazepam in benzodiazepine dependence. *British Journal of Psychiatry*, **158**, 511–516.

Nagy, L.M., Krystal, J.H., Woods, S.W., & Charney, D.S. (1989). Clinical and medication outcome after short-term alprazolam and behavioral group treatment in panic disorder. 2.5 year naturalistic follow-up study. *Archives of General Psychiatry*, **46**, 993–999.

Nordentoft, M., Breum, L., Munck, L., Nordestgaard, A.G., Hunding, A., & Laursen Bjældager, P.A. (1993). High mortality by natural and unnnatural causes: a 10-year follow-up study of patients admitted to a poisoning treatment centre after suicide attempts. *British Medical Journal,* **306**, 1637–1641.

Noyes, R., Reich, J., Christiansen, J., *et al.* (1980). Outcome of panic disorder, relationship to diagnostic subtypes and comorbidity. *Archives of General Psychiatry,* **47**, 809–818.

Noyes, R. Jr., Anderson, D.J., Clancy, J., Crowe, R.R., Slymen, D.J., Ghoneim, M.M., & Hinrichs, J.V. (1984). Diazepam and propranolol in panic disorder and agoraphobia. *Archives of General Psychiatry,* **41**, 287–292.

Noyes, R.J., Woodman, C.L., Holt, C.S., Reich, J.H., & Zimmerman, M.B. (1995). Avoidant personality traits distinguish social phobic and panic disorder subjects. *Journal of Nervous and Mental Disease,* **183**, 145–153.

Oldham, J.M., Skodol, A.E., Kellman, H.D., Hyler, S.E., Doidge, N., Rosnick, L., & Gallaher, P.E. (1995). Comorbidity of axis I and axis II disorders. *American Journal of Psychiatry,* **152**, 571–578.

Ormel, J., Oldehinkel, T., Brilman, E., & Brink, W.V. (1993). Outcome of depression and anxiety in primary care: a three wave 3½ year study of psychopathology and disability. *Archives of General Psychiatry,* **50**, 759–767.

Osler, W. (1912). *The Principles and Practice of Medicine,* 8th edition. pp. 1108–1109. London: Appleton.

Ost, L.G., Westling, B.E., & Hellstrom, K. (1993). Applied relaxation, exposure in vivo and cognitive methods in the treatment of panic disorder with agoraphobia. *Behaviour Research and Therapy,* **31**, 383–394.

Otto, M.W., Pollack, M.H., Sachs, G.S., Reiter, S.R., Meltzer Brody, S., & Rosenbaum, J.F. (1993). Discontinuation of benzodiazepine treatment: efficacy of cognitive-behavioral therapy for patients with panic disorder. *American Journal of Psychiatry,* **150**, 1485–1490.

Payne, A., & Blanchard, E.B. (1995). A controlled comparison of cognitive therapy and self-help support groups in the treatment of irritable bowel syndrome. *Journal of Consulting and Clinical Psychology,* **63**, 779–786.

Perry, J.C., Lavori, P.W., & Hoke, L. (1987). A Markov model for prediction levels of psychiatric service use in borderline and antisocial personality disorders and bipolar type II affective disorder. *Journal of Psychiatric Research*, **21**, 215–232.

Perse, T.L., Greist, J.H., Jefferson, J.W., Rosenfeldt, R., & Dar, R. (1987). Fluvoxamine treatment of obsessive-compulsive disorder. *American Journal of Psychiatry*, **144**, 1543–1548.

Pigott, T.A., L'Heureux, F., Dubbert, B., Bernstein, S., & Murphy, D.L. (1994). Obsessive compulsive disorder: comorbid conditions. *Journal of Clinical Psychiatry (Suppl)*, **55**, 15–27.

Pollack, M.H., Otto, M.W., Sachs, G.S., Leon, A., Shear, M.K., Deltito, J.A., Keller, M.B., & Rosenbaum, J.F. (1994). Anxiety psychopathology predictive of outcome in patients with panic disorder and depression treated with imipramine, alprazolam and placebo. *Journal of Affective Disorders*, **30**, 273–281.

Power, K.G., Jerrom, D.W.A., Simpson, R.J., & Mitchell, M. (1985). Controlled study of withdrawal symptoms and rebound anxiety after six week course of diazepam for generalised anxiety. *British Medical Journal*, **290**, 1246–1248.

Power, K.G., Simpson, R.J., Swanson, V., & Wallace, L.A. (1990). Controlled comparison of pharmacological and psychological treatment of generalized anxiety disorder in primary care. *British Journal of General Practice*, **40**, 289–294.

Puccinelli, M., & Wilkinson, G. (1994). Outcome of depression in psychiatric settings. *British Journal of Psychiatry*, **164**, 297–304.

Quinton, D., Gulliver, L., & Rutter, M. (1995). A 15–20 year follow-up of adult psychiatric patients. Psychiatric disorder and social functioning. *British Journal of Psychiatry*, **167**, 315–323.

Ramsay, R. (1990). Invited review: post-traumatic stress disorder; a new clinical entity? *Journal of Psychomatic Research*, **34**, 355–365.

Rasch, G. (1960). Probabilistic models for some intelligence and attainment tests. Copenhagen: Danish Institute of Education and Research.

Ravaris, C.L., Nies, A., Robinson, D.S., Ives, J.O., & Bartlett, D. (1976). A multiple-dose controlled study of phenelzine in depressive-anxiety states. *Archives of General Psychiatry*, **33**, 347–350.

Regier, D.A., Narrow, W.E., & Rae, D.S. (1990a). The epidemiology of anxiety disorders: the Epidemiologic Catchment Area (ECA) experience. *Journal of Psychiatric Research (Suppl 2)*, **24**, 3–14.

Regier, D.A., Farmer, M.E., Rae, D.S., Locke, B.Z., Keith, S.J., Judd, L.L., & Goodwin, F.K. (1990b). Comorbidity of mental disorders with alcohol and other drug abuse. Results from the Epidemiologic Catchment Area (ECA) Study. *Journal of the American Medical Association*, **264**, 2511–2518.

Regier, D.A., Rae, D.S., Narrow, W.E., Kaelber, C.T., & Schatzberg, A.F. (1998). The prevalence of anxiety disorders and their comorbidity with mood and addictive disorders. *British Journal of Psychiatry (Suppl 34)*, **173**, 24–28.

Reich, J.H., & Vasile, R.G. (1993). Effect of personality disorders on the treatment outcome of axis I conditions: an update. *Journal of Nervous and Mental Disease*, **181**, 475–484.

Reiman, E.M., Raichle, M.E., Butler, F.K., Herscovitch, P., & Robins, E. (1985). A focal brain abnormality in panic disorder, a severe form of anxiety. *Nature*, **310**, 683–685.

Rice, K.M., & Blanchard, E.B. (1982). Biofeedback in the treatment of anxiety disorders. *Clinical Psychological Review*, **2**, 557–577.

Robins, L.N., Wing, J., Wittchen, H.U., Helzer, J.E., Babor, T.F., Burke, J., Farmer, A., Jablenski, A., Pickens, R., Regier, D.A., *et al.* (1988). The Composite International Diagnostic Interview. An epidemiologic instrument suitable for use in conjunction with different diagnostic systems and in different cultures. *Archives of General Psychiatry*, **45**, 1069–1077.

Roth, M., & Argyle, N. (1988). Anxiety, panic and phobic disorders: an overview. *Journal of Psychiatric Research (Suppl 1)*, **22**, 33–54.

Rotter, J.B. (1966). Generalised expectancies for internal versus external control of reinforcement. *Psychological Monographs*, **80**, 609.

Rounsaville, B.J., Anton, S.F., Carroll, K., Budde, D., Prusoff, B.A. & Gawin, F. (1991). Psychiatric diagnoses of treatment-seeking cocaine abusers. *Archiver of General Psychiatry*, **48**, 43–51.

Roy, M.A., Neale, M.C., Pedersen, N.L., Mathe, A.A., & Kendler, K.S. (1995). A twin study of generalized anxiety disorder and major depression. *Psychological Medicine*, **25**, 1037–1049.

Roy-Byrne, P.P., & Cowley, D.S. (1995). Course and outcome of panic disorder: a review of recent follow-up studies. *Anxiety*, **1**, 151–160.

Rush, C.R., & Griffiths, R.R. (1996). Zolpidem, triazolam, and temazepam: behavioral and subject-rated effects in normal volunteers. *Journal of Clinical Psychopharmacology*, **16**, 146–157.

Rutter, M. (1985). Resilience in the face of adversity. *British Journal of Psychiatry*, **147**, 598–611.

Rutter, M. (1987). Temperament, personality and personality disorder. *British Journal of Psychiatry*, **150**, 443–458.

Sackett, D.L., Rosenberg, W.M., Gray, J.A., Haynes, R.B., & Richardson, W.S. (1996). Evidence based medicine: what is it and what it isn't. *British Medical Journal*, **312**, 71–72.

Salkovskis, P.M., Clark, D.M., & Hackmann, A. (1991). Treatment of panic attacks using cognitive therapy without exposure or breathing retraining. *Behaviour Research and Therapy*, **29**, 161–166.

Schapira, K., Roth, M., Kerr, T.A., & Gurney, C. (1972). The prognosis of affective disorders: the differentiation of anxiety states from depressive illnesses. *British Journal of Psychiatry*, **121**, 175–181.

Schneier, F.R., Heckelman, L.R., Garfinkel, R., Campeas, R., Fallon, B.A., Gitow, A., Street, L., Del Bene, D., & Liebowitz, M.R. (1994). Functional impairment in social phobia. *Journal of Clinical Psychiatry*, **55**, 322–331.

Seivewright, H., Tyrer, P., & Johnson, T. (1998). Prediction of outcome in neurotic disorder: a 5-year prospective study. *Psychological Medicine*, **28**, 1149–1157.

Seivewright, N. (1987). Relationship between life events and personality in psychiatric disorder. *Stress Medicine*, **3**, 163–168.

Seligman, M.E.P. (1975). *Helplessness: On Depression, Development and Death*. San Francisco: Freeman.

Shapiro, F. (1989). Eye movement desensitization: a new treatment for post-traumatic stress disorder. *Journal of Behaviour Therapy and Experiential Psychiatry*, **20**, 211–217.

Shea, M.T., Pilkonis, P.A., Beckham, E., Collins, J.F., Elkin, I., Sotsky, S.M., & Docherty, J.P. (1990). Personality disorders and treatment outcome in the NIMH Treatment of Depression Collaborative Research Program. *American Journal of Psychiatry*, **147**, 711–718.

Shea, M.T., Elkin, I., Imber, S.D., Sotsky, S.M., Watkins, J.T., Collins, J.F., Pilkonis, P.A., Beckham, E., Glass, D.R., Dolan, R.T., *et al.* (1992). Course of depressive symptoms over follow-up. Findings from the National Institute of Mental Health Treatment of Depression Collaborative Research Program. *Archives of General Psychiatry*, **49**, 782–787.

Sheehan, D.V. (1983). *The Anxiety Disease*. New York: Charles Scribner's Sons.

Sheehan, D.V., Raj, A.B., Harnett-Sheehan, K., Soto, S., & Knapp, E. (1993). The relative efficacy of high-dose buspirone and alprazolam in the treatment of panic disorder: a double-blind placebo-controlled study. *Acta Psychiatrica Scandinavica*, **88**, 1–11.

Sherbourne, C.D., Jackson, C.A., Meredith, L.S., Camp, P., & Wells, K.B. (1996). Prevalence of comorbid anxiety disorders in primary care outpatients. *Archives of Family Medicine*, **5**, 27–34.

Simon, G.E., & VonKorff, M. (1991). Somatization and psychiatric disorder in the NIMH Epidemiologic Catchment Area study. *American Journal of Psychiatry*, **148**, 1494–1500.

Skinner, B.F. (1938). *The Behavior of Organisms*. New York: Appleton-Century-Crofts.

Smith, W.P., Compton, W.C., & West, W.B. (1995). Meditation as an adjunct to a happiness enhancement program. *Journal of Clinical Psychology*, **51**, 269–273.

Snaith, R.P., Constanopoulos, A.A., Jardine, M.Y., & McGuffin, P. (1978). A clinical scale for the self-assessment of irritability, anxiety and depression. *British Journal of Psychiatry*, **132**, 164–167.

Snaith, R.P., Baugh, S.J., Clayden, A.D., Hussain, A., & Sipple, M.A. (1982). The Clinical Anxiety Scale: an instrument derived from the Hamilton Anxiety Scale. *British Journal of Psychiatry*, **141**, 518–523.

Spielberger, C.D., Gorsuch, R.L., & Lushene, R.E. (1968). *Manual for the State-Trait Anxiety Inventory*. Tallahassee: Florida State University.

Spitzer, R.L., & Williams, J.B.W. (1995). *Structured Clinical Interview for DSM-IV-Patient Version (SCID-P)*. New York: Biometrics Research Department, New York State Psychiatric Institute.

Starcevic, V., Fallon, S., Uhlenhuth, E.H., & Pathak, D. (1994). Comorbidity rates do not support distinction between panic disorder and generalised anxiety disorder. *Psychopathology*, **27**, 269–272.

Starcevic, V., Uhlenhuth, E.H., Kellner, R., & Pathak, D. (1993). Comparison of primary and secondary panic disorder: a preliminary report. *Journal of Affective Disorders*, **27**, 81–86.

Suinn, R., & Richardson, F. (1971). Anxiety management training: a non-specific behavior therapy program for anxiety control. *Behavior Therapy*, **2**, 498–511.

Surtees, P.G., & Barkley, C. (1994). Future imperfect: the long-term outcome of depressive disorder. *British Journal of Psychiatry*, **164**, 327–341.

Taylor, C.B., Kenigsberg, M.L., & Robinson, J.M. (1982). A controlled comparison of relaxation and diazepam in panic disorder. *Journal of Clinical Psychiatry*, **43**, 423–425.

Taylor, J.A. (1953). A personality scale of manifest anxiety. *Journal of Abnormal and Social Psychology*, **48**, 285–295.

Thompson, A.H., Bland, R.C., & Orn, H.T. (1989). Relationship and chronology of depression, agoraphobia, and panic disorder in the general population. *Journal of Nervous and Mental Disease*, **177**, 456–463.

Thorndike, E.L. (1911). *Animal Intelligence*. New York: Macmillan.

Trethowan, W.H. (1975). Pills for personal problems. *British Medical Journal*, **iii**, 749–751.

Tye, N.C., Everitt, B.J., & Iversen, S.D. (1977). 5-Hydroxytryptamine and the punishment. *Nature (London)*, **268**, 741–742.

Tyrer, P. (1985). Neurosis divisible? *Lancet*, **i**, 685–688.

Tyrer, P., & Casey, P. (1993). *Social Function in Psychiatry: The Hidden Axis of Classification Exposed*. Petersfield: Wrightson Biomedical Publishing Ltd.

Tyrer, P., & Seivewright, H. (1988). Studies of outcome. In: *Personality Disorders: Diagnosis, Management and Course* (ed. Tyrer, P.), pp. 119–136. London: Butterworth (Wright).

Tyrer, P., & Hallström, C. (1993). Antidepressants in the treatment of anxiety disorder. *Psychiatric Bulletin*, **17**, 75–76.

Tyrer, P., & Steinberg, D. (1998). *Models for Mental Disorder. Conceptual Models in Psychiatry, 3rd edition.* Chichester: John Wiley.

Tyrer, P. (1974). The benzodiazepine bonanza. *Lancet*, **ii**, 709–710.

Tyrer, P. (1980). Dependence on benzodiazepines. *British Journal of Psychiatry*, **137**, 576–577.

Tyrer, P. (1982). The concept of somatic anxiety. *British Journal of Psychiatry*, **140**, 325.

Tyrer, P. (1984). Clinical effects of abrupt withdrawal from tri-cyclic antidepressants and monoamine oxidase inhibitors after long-term treatment. *Journal of Affective Disorders*, **6**, 1–7.

Tyrer, P. (1986). *How to Stop Taking Tranquillisers.* London: Sheldon Press.

Tyrer, P., Ferguson, B., Fowler-Dixon, R., & Kelemen, A. (1990a). A plea for the diagnosis of hypochondriacal personality disorder. *Journal of Psychosomatic Research*, **34**, 637–642.

Tyrer, P. (1990b). The division of neurosis: a failed classification. *Journal of the Royal Society of Medicine*, **83**, 614–616.

Tyrer, P. (1991). The nocebo effect — Poorly known but getting stronger. In: *Side Effects of Drugs Annual 15* (eds. Dukes, M.N.G., & Aronson, J.K.), pp. 19–25. Amsterdam: Elsevier.

Tyrer, P. (1992a). Anxiety and depression: a clinical profile. In: *Experimental Approaches to Anxiety and Depression* (eds. Elliott, D.J., & Marsden, C.A.), pp. 9–25. Chichester: John Wiley & Sons.

Tyrer, P. (1992b). Anxiolytics not acting at the benzodiazepine receptor: beta blockers. *Progress in Neuro-Psychopharmacology and Biological Psychiatry*, **16**, 17–26.

Tyrer, P. (1994). Anxiety disorder. In: *Prevention in Psychiatry* (eds. Paykel, E.S., & Jenkins, R.), pp. 88–95. London: Gaskell Books, Royal College of Psychiatrists.

Tyrer, P. (1995). Are personality disorders well described in DSM-IV? In: *The DSM-IV personality disorders*, (ed. Livesley, W.J.), New York: Guilford Press.

Tyrer, P. (1996). Comorbidity or consanguinity. *British Journal of Psychiatry*, **168**, 669–671.

Tyrer, P. (1999) (ed.). *Personality Disorders: Diagnosis, Management and Course, 2nd edition*. London: Butterworth-Heinemann.

Tyrer, P., Casey, P., & Ferguson, B. (1988a). Personality disorder and mental illness. In: *Personality Disorders: Diagnosis, Management and Course* (ed. Tyrer, P.), pp. 93–104. London: Butterworth (Wright).

Tyrer, P., Seivewright, N., Ferguson, B., Murphy, S., Darling, C., Brothwell, J., Kingdon, D., Johnson, A.L. (1990b). The Nottingham study of neurotic disorder: relationship between personality status and symptoms. *Psychological Medicine*, **20**, 423–431.

Tyrer, P., Seivewright, N., Murphy, S., Ferguson, B., Kingdon, D., Brothwell. J., Darling, C., Barczak, P., Gregory, S., & Johnson, A.L. (1988b). The Nottingham study of neurotic disorder: comparison of drug and psychological treatments. *Lancet*, **ii**, 235–240.

Tyrer, P., Seivewright, N., Ferguson, B., Murphy, S., & Johnson, A.L. (1993). The Nottingham study of neurotic disorder: effect of personality status on response to drug treatment, cognitive therapy and self help over two years. *British Journal of Psychiatry*, **162**, 219–226.

Tyrer, P., Marsden, C., Ferguson, B., Murphy, S., Hannon, S., & Greenwood, D. (1991). Clinical and humoral effects of beta-blockade with ICI 118,551 in the general neurotic syndrome. *Journal of Psychopharmacology*, **5**, 238–242.

Tyrer, P., & Lader, M. (1972). Beta-adrenergic-receptor blockade in the treatment of anxiety. *The Lancet*, **2**, 542.

Tyrer, P., & Murphy, S. (1987). The place of benzodiazepines in psychiatric practice. *British Journal of Psychiatry*, **151**, 719–723.

Tyrer, P., & Alexander, J. (1979). Classification of personality disorder. *British Journal of Psychiatry*, **135**, 163–167.

Tyrer, P., & Johnson, T. (1996). Establishing the severity of personality disorder. *American Journal of Psychiatry*, **153**, 1593–1597.

Tyrer, P., & Tyrer, J. (1993). Antidepressive drugs for the treatment of anxiety disorders and vice versa. In: *Handbook on Depression and Anxiety: A Biological Approach* (ed. den Boer, J.A., & Sitsen, A.B.), pp. 497–515. Amsterdam: Elsevier.

Tyrer, P., Candy, J., & Kelly, D. (1973). A study of the clinical effects of phenelzine and placebo in the treatment of phobic anxiety. *Psychopharmacologia*, **32**, 237–254.

Tyrer, P., Cicchetti, D.V., Casey, P.R., Fitzpatrick, K., Oliver, R., Balter, A., Giller, E., & Harkness, L. (1984). Cross-national reliability study of a schedule for assessing personality disorders. *Journal of Nervous and Mental Diseases*, **172**, 718–721.

Tyrer, P., Ferguson, B., Hallstrom, C., Michie, M., Tyrer, S., Cooper, S., Caplan, R., & Barczak, P. (1996). A controlled trial of dothiepin and placebo in treating benzodiazepine withdrawal symptoms. *British Journal of Psychiatry*, **168**, 457–461.

Tyrer, P., Gunderson, J., Lyons, M., & Tohen, M. (1997a). Extent of comorbidity between mental state and personality disorders. *Journal of Personality Disorders*, **11**, 242–259.

Tyrer, P., Harrison-Read, P., & Van Horn, E. (1997b). *Drug Treatment in Psychiatry: A Guide for the Community Health Worker.* Oxford: Butterworth-Heinemann.

Tyrer, P., Horn, S., & Lee, I. (1978). Treatment of agoraphobia by subliminal and supraliminal exposure to phobic cine film. *Lancet*, **1**, 358–360.

Tyrer, P., Lee, I., & Alexander, J. (1980). Awareness of cardiac function in anxious, phobic and hypochondriacal patients. *Psychological Medicine*, **10**, 171–174.

Tyrer, P., Murphy, S., Oates, G., & Kingdon, D. (1985). Psychological treatment for benzodiazepine dependence. *The Lancet*, **1**, 1042–1043.

Tyrer, P., Owen, R., & Dawling, S. (1983). Gradual withdrawal of diazepam after long-term therapy. *Lancet*, **i**, 1402–1406.

Tyrer, P., Owen, R.T., & Cicchetti, D. (1984). The brief scale for anxiety: a subdivision of the Comprehensive Psychopathological Rating Scale. *Journal of Neurology, Neurosurgery and Psychiatry*, **47**, 970–975.

Tyrer, P., Seivewright, N., Ferguson, B., & Tyrer, J. (1992). The general neurotic syndrome: a coaxial diagnosis of anxiety, depression and personality disorder. *Acta Psychiatrica Scandinavica*, **85**, 201–206.

Tyrer, P.J., & Kasriel, J. (1975). Genetical components of physiological tremor. *Journal of Medical Genetics*, **12**, 162–164.

Tyrer, P.J., & Lader, M.H. (1974). Tremor in acute and chronic anxiety. *Archives of General Psychiatry*, **31**, 506–509.

Tyrer, P.J. (1973a). Relevance of bodily feelings in emotion. *Lancet*, **i**, 915–916.

Tyrer, P.J. (1973b). Are monoamine-oxidase inhibitors antidepressants? *Proceedings of the Royal Society of Medicine*, **66**, 950–951.

Tyrer, P.J., & Lader, M.H. (1973). Effects of beta adrenergic blockade with sotalol in chronic anxiety. *Clinical Pharmacology and Therapeutics*, **14**, 418–426.

Tyrer, P.J., & Lader, M.H. (1976). Central and peripheral correlates of anxiety: a comparative study. *Journal of Nervous and Mental Disease*, **162**, 99–104.

Uhrbrand, L., & Faurbye, A. (1960). Reversible and irreversible dyskinesia after treatment with perphenazine, chlorpromazine, reserpine and electroconvulsive therapy. *Psychopharmacologia*, **1**, 408–419.

Vaglum, S., & Vaglum, P. (1989). Comorbidity for borderline and schizotypal personality disorders. A study of alcoholic women. *Journal of Nervous and Mental Disease*, **177**, 279–284.

Van Ameringen, M., Mancini, C., Styan, G., & Donison, D. (1991). Relationship of social phobia with other psychiatric illness. *Journal of Affective Disorders*, **21**, 93–99.

Van Balkom, A.J., Bakker, A., Spinhoven, P., Blaauw, B.M., Smeenk, S., & Ruesink, B. (1997). A meta-analysis of the treatment of panic disorder with or without agoraphobia: a comparison of psychopharmacological, cognitive-behavioral, and combination treatments. *Journal of Nervous and Mental Disease*, **185**, 510–516.

Van den Hout, M., Arntz, A., & Hoekstra, R. (1994). Exposure reduced agoraphobia but not panic, and cognitive therapy reduced panic but not agoraphobia. *Behaviour Research and Therapy*, **32**, 447–451.

Van Valkenburg, C., Akiskal, H.S., Puzantian, V., & Rosenthal, T. (1984). Anxious depressions: clinical, family history, and naturalistic outcome — Comparisons with panic and major depressive disorders. *Journal of Affective Disorders*, **6**, 67–82.

Versiani, M., Nardi, A.E., Mundim, F.D., Alves, A.B., Liebowitz, M.R., and Amrein, R. (1992). Pharmacotherapy of social phobia. A controlled study with moclobemide and phenelzine. *British Journal of Psychiatry*, **161**, 353–360.

Vollrath, M., & Angst, J. (1989). Outcome of panic and depression in a seven year follow-up: Results of the Zurich study. *Acta Psychiatria Scandinavica*, **80**, 591–596.

Warshaw, M.G., Keller, M.B., & Stout, R.L. (1994). Reliability and validity of the longitudinal interval follow-up evaluation for assessing outcome of anxiety disorders. *Journal of Psychiatric Research*, **28**, 531–545.

Warwick, H.M. (1989). A cognitive-behavioural approach to hypochondriasis and health anxiety. *Journal of Psychosomatic Research*, **33**, 705–711.

Watson, J.P., Gaind, R., & Marks, I.M. (1972). Physiological habituation to continuous phobic stimulation. *Behaviour Research and Therapy*, **20**, 269–278.

Weekes, C. (1962). *Self Help for Your Nerves*. London: Angus & Robertson.

Weissman, M.M. (1985). The epidemiology of anxiety disorders: rates, risks and familial patterns. In: *Anxiety and the Anxiety Disorders* (eds. Tuma, A.H., & Maser, J.D.), Hillsdale, New Jersey: Erlbaum Associates.

Welkowitz, L.A., Papp, L.A., Cloitre, M., Liebowitz, M.R., Martin, L.Y., & Gorman, J.M. (1991). Cognitive-behavior therapy for panic disorder delivered by psychopharmacologically oriented clinicians. *Journal of Nervous and Mental Disease*, **179**, 473–477.

Wells, K.B., Golding, J.M., & Burnam, M.A. (1989). Chronic medical conditions in a sample of the general population with anxiety, affective, and substance use disorders. *American Journal of Psychiatry*, **146**, 1440–1446.

Wessely, S., Chalder, T., Hirsch, S., Wallace, P., & Wright, D. (1996). Psychological symptoms, somatic symptoms, and psychiatric disorder in chronic fatigue and chronic fatigue syndrome: a prospective study in the primary care setting. *American Journal of Psychiatry*, **153**, 1050–1059.

Westphal, C. (1871). Die Agoraphobie: eine neuropathische Eischeinung. *Archives für Psychiatrie und Nervenkrankheiten*, **3**, 384–412.

Wiborg, I.M., & Dahl, A.A. (1996). Does brief dynamic psychotherapy reduce the relapse rate of panic disorder? *Archives of General Psychiatry*, **53**, 689–694.

Wing, J.K., Cooper, J., & Sartorius, N. (1974). *The Measurement and Classification of Psychiatric Symptoms*. Cambridge: Cambridge University Press.

Winokur, G. (1990). The concept of secondary depression and its relationship to comorbidity. *Psychiatric Clinics of North America*, **13**, 567–583.

Wittchen, H.U., & Essau, C.A. (1993). Comorbidity and mixed anxiety-depressive disorders: is there epidemiologic evidence? *Journal of Clinical Psychiatry (Suppl)*, **54**, 9–15.

Wolpe, J. (1958). *Psychotherapy By Reciprocal Inhibition*. Stanford: Stanford University Press.

Woodruff, R., Murphy, G., & Herjanic, M. (1967). The natural history of affective disorders: 1 — Symptoms of 72 patients at the time of index hospital admission. *Journal of Psychiatric Research*, **5**, 255–263.

World Health Organisation (1992). *International Classification of Diseseases, 10th revision*. Geneva: World Health Organisation.

World Psychiatric Association Dysthymia Working Group (1995). Dysthymia in clinical practice. *British Journal of Psychiatry*, **166**, 174–183.

Yerkes, R.M., & Dodson, J.D. (1908). The relation of strength of stimulus to rapidity of habit-formation. *Journal of Comparative Neurology and Psychology*, **18**, 459–482.

Yonkers, K.A. (1997). Anxiety symptoms and anxiety disorders: how are they related to premenstrual disorders? *Journal of Clinical Psychiatry (Suppl 3)*, **58**, 62–67.

Young, J.P.R., Fenton, G.W., & Lader, M.H. (1971). Inheritance of neurotic traits: a twin study of the Middlesex Hospital Questionnaire. *British Journal of Psychiatry*, **119**, 393–398.

Young, J.P.R., Hughes, W.C., & Lader, M.H. (1976). A controlled comparison of flupenthixol and amitriptyline in depressed outpatients. *British Medical Journal,* 1, 1116–1118.

Zajecka, J., Tracy, K.A., & Mitchell, S. (1997). Discontinuation symptoms after treatment with serotonin reuptake inhibitors: a literature review. *Journal of Clinical Psychiatry,* 58, 291–297.

Zigmond, A.S., & Snaith, R.P. (1983). The Hospital Anxiety and Depression Scale. *Acta Psychiatrica Scandinavica,* 57, 361–370.

Zinbarg, R.E., Barlow, D.H., Liebowitz, M., Street, L., Broadhead, E., Katon, W., Roy Byrne, P., Lepine, J.P., Teherani, M., Richards, J., *et al.* (1994). The DSM-IV field trial for mixed anxiety-depression. *American Journal of Psychiatry,* 151, 1153–1162.

Zitrin, C.M., Klein, D.F., Woerner, N.G., & Ross, D.C. (1983). Treatment of phobias. 1. Comparison of imipramine hydrochloride and placebo. *Archives of General Psychiatry,* 40, 125–138.

Acknowledgement page for book on Anxiety

Acknowledgements following for permission to reproduce material in this book; the World Health Organisation and American Psychiatric Association, for diagnostic criteria for neurotic disorders from the *International Classification of Diseases* and the *Diagnostic and Statistical Manual for Mental Disorders*, Dr Philip Snaith for the Hospital Anxiety and Depression Scale, the Clinical Anxiety Scale and the Irritability, Depression and Anxiety Scale, the *Journal of Neurology, Neurosurgery and Psychiatry* for the Brief Anxiety Scale, Professors Isaac Marks and Andrew Mathews for the Fear Questionnaire and the Phobia Scale (Figure 2.9), *Clinical Pharmacology and Therapeutics* for Figure 2.11, *Psychological Medicine* for Figure 4.6, Oxford University Press for Figure 4.4, Professors Goldberg and Huxley and Tavistock/Routledge for Figure 5.2, the *British Journal of Psychiatry* for Figure 8.2, John Wiley & Sons for Table 9.5, and *Acta Psychiatrica Scandinavica* for Figure 9.2.

INDEX

C

L

M

S